Oddly
Enough

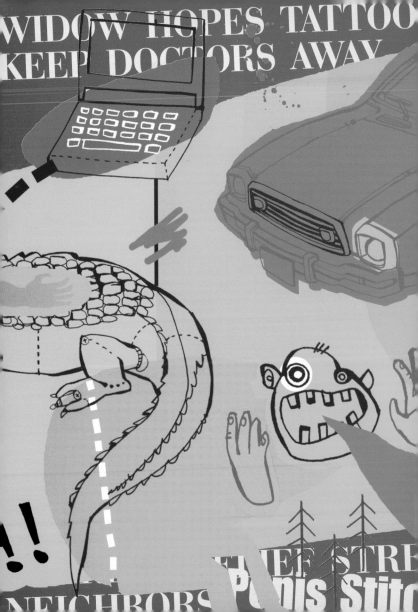

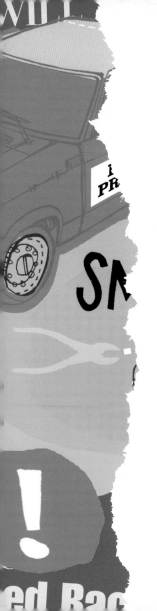

Oddly Enough

edited by
ROBERT BASLER

REUTERS

MQP

PUBLISHED BY **MQ Publications Limited**
12 The Ivories
6–8 Northampton Street
London, N1 2HY
EMAIL: mqpublications.com
WEBSITE: www.mqpublications.com

COPYRIGHT © 2004 MQ Publications Limited
TEXT COPYRIGHT © 2004 **Reuters**

DESIGN CONCEPT **Balley Design Associates**

ISBN: 1-84072-595-8

10 9 8 7 6 5 4 3 2 1

Printed and bound in Italy

Contents

Foreword

GUARANTEE
SEX EVERY
NIGHT

A parachutist lands on a beer vendor at a coleslaw wrestling match. Two social workers visit a client in her apartment, then leave, never realizing that she is dead. An aging playboy finds an ingenious way to guarantee sex every night. A young woman in London lets a stranger smear her feet with baked beans…

Welcome to the kind of stories they don't give Pulitzer Prizes for, but probably should.

As I write this foreword, Washington has just confirmed that Saddam Hussein survived the Iraq war, and a tropical storm is poised to strike the U.S. Gulf Coast. It is a huge news day, and what is the most-read news story on Yahoo's Internet site? A piece headlined "Blunder Leaves Woman Awake During Surgery."

Journalists call such stories "brights"—a misnomer indeed, since many of these items are dark, tragic, grotesque and tasteless. Whatever we call them, they have one thing in common: the good ones have a truly universal appeal.

Let's back up for a moment. Reuters, a news agency with more than 150 years of history, is among the most serious and respected news organizations in the world. Our reporters, photographers and cameramen go everywhere, covering the toughest assignments and are no strangers to great personal risk. Indeed, too many have given their lives to cover the news.

…This is the news remember

FOREWORD...
2,400 journalists

Every day we count our headlines in the tens of thousands and our words in the millions. Our news goes to investors, newspapers, broadcasters and Web sites. It informs governments and is essential to traders in the world's financial markets.

And it turns out, when you have more than 2,400 journalists in nearly 200 far-flung bureaus covering big, important stories, they're also going to find some great little, less important ones as well. We use these in a popular daily product called *Oddly Enough*, and the book you're holding is a collection of the very best of them from the past few years.

Why are brights so popular? I think we take great pleasure in knowing that these things didn't happen to us and aren't likely to. Our daily news is filled with details that worry us and weigh us down, but hey! The chances are fairly slim that a parachutist is going to land on me while I'm watching a coleslaw wrestling match. To me, as a reader, that sounds like a pretty good deal.

So, settle back with this book and read all about the voodoo latrine, the long doughnut trail, the insurance scam chainsaw horror... This is the news you'll remember when you want to forget everything else.

Robert Basler
Global Online Editor | REUTERS

COLESLAW
WRESTLING
MATCH

ou'll

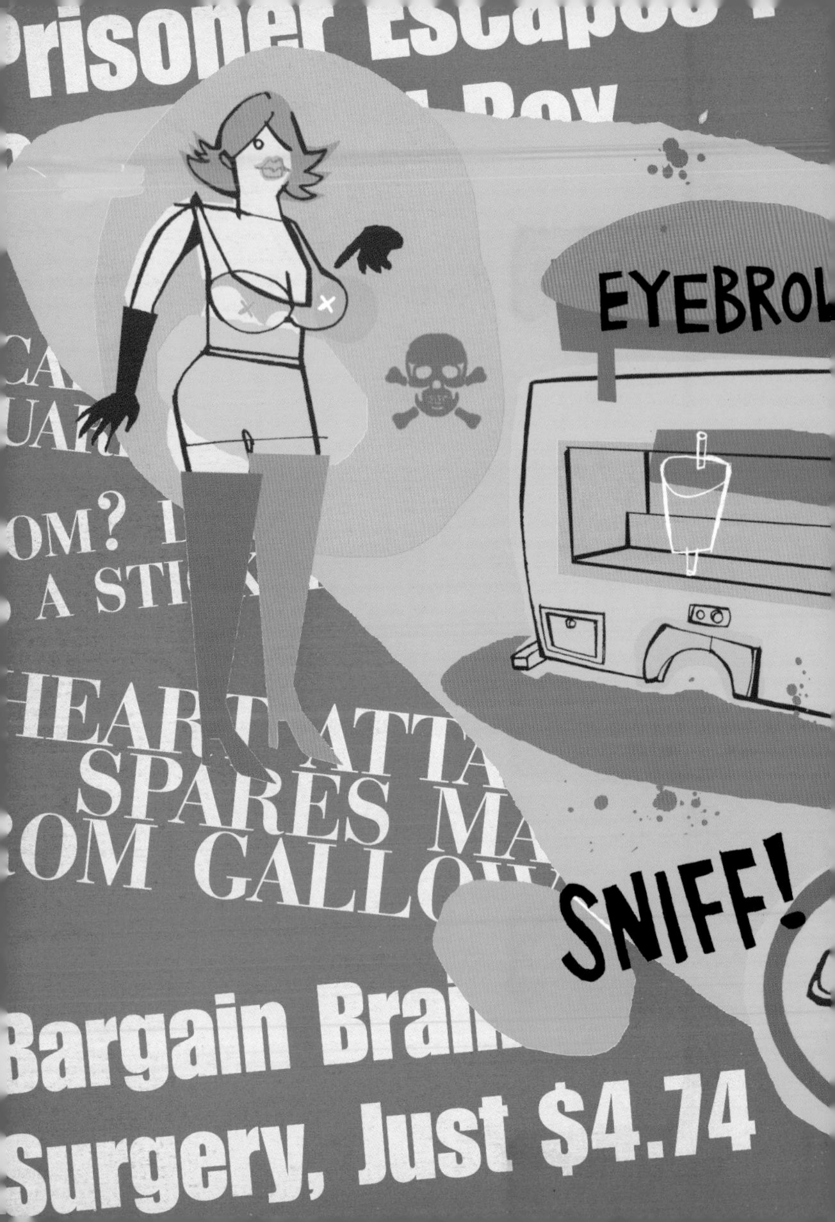
EYEBRO
SPARES MA
OM GALLO
SNIFF!
Bargain Bra
Surgery, Just $4.74

CHAPTER 1

It's Not Brain Surgery...

KEBABS

$4.74

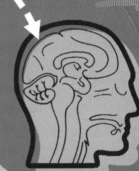

fetish.com

Bargain Brain Surgery, Just $4.74

CAIRO — REUTERS

Egyptian police have arrested a man who performed brain surgery on a number of people although he had only a primary school education, court sources said.

The 40-year-old man saw around 200 patients a week in the oasis town of Fayoum near Cairo. He charged 22 Egyptian pounds ($4.74) per patient and operated on a number of people but the fate of his victims was not immediately known.

The man had forged a secondary school certificate and claimed to have studied brain surgery in Cairo and Germany.

HEART ATTACK SPARES MAN FROM GALLOWS

TEHRAN — REUTERS

A convicted Iranian murderer cheated death when he was spared from a public hanging because he had a heart attack after the noose was placed around his neck, newspapers said.

Mohammad Hadi, a 55-year-old drug dealer convicted of killing one of his customers last year, had the narrow escape from death just before his execution in the main square of the central city Khomeini Shahr.

But Hadi's reprieve is only temporary. He has been transferred to a hospital for treatment and once he recovers his execution will be carried out as planned, the *Qods* daily said.

Bank Robbed By Its Own Guard

JERUSALEM   REUTERS

An Israeli bank was robbed at gunpoint by its own security guard, who made off with 100,000 shekels ($21,000), police said.

A police spokesman said he expected police to catch the guard soon because "we know everything about him."

The guard was employed by a security company that has a contract with Bank Leumi, Israel's second largest bank, a spokeswoman said.

She said the guard went into the Leumi branch in the Tel Aviv suburb of Petah Tikva after the bank closed to customers but bank employees were still working, and he told a teller to give him the money.

She said the bank was currently investigating the incident with the security company, whose guards are licensed to carry weapons.

VOODOO LATRINE

KINGSTON | Jamaica   REUTERS

A musical greeting card tinkled out the tune to "Silent Night" from the depths of a Jamaican latrine, prompting a voodoo scare that led to a cache of missing mail, the Caribbean News Agency reported.

The musical card was among hundreds of letters found dumped into the post office latrine in Kingston's Grove Town community, the agency said.

The letters were discovered on December 19, when a man using the pit-style latrine heard the instrumental version of "Silent Night" ringing up from the depths of the facility.

Believing he was the victim of a voodoo curse, the frightened man alerted neighbors, who searched the latrine and discovered the undelivered mail, the agency said.

Police were still investigating how the mail ended up in the latrine.

Jewelry Thieves Suck

PARIS   REUTERS

Thieves behind a rash of daring jewelry heists in Paris have used a bewildering variety of tactics to snatch their precious haul, but the latest innovation, a vacuum cleaner, has surprised even the police.

Four men on motorcycles roared up to a jewelers in a wealthy Paris district, smashed glass display units and then used a battery-operated, hand-held vacuum to clean up.

"Thieves certainly don't lack innovation," said Patrick Mauduit, a spokesman for police officers' union Synergie Officiers.

"In one swipe they sucked up jewels that usually have to be picked by hand."

Mom? Dad? It's A Stickup

STOCKHOLM   REUTERS

A 27-year-old Swede was charged with taking part in the armed robbery of his own parents, during which his mother was shot in the arm.

The man is accused of breaking into his parents' house in Eskilstuna, west of Stockholm, with six accomplices. They stole money and a number of valuables thought to be worth over one million crowns ($124,200), according to the prosecution filing to the court.

It said the man, who has a history of drug abuse, first told police he had been taken hostage by the gang and tied up after they entered the house, but evidence from taped telephone conversations disproved his claims.

GUNS DON'T KILL PEOPLE—UMBRELLAS DO

TOKYO   REUTERS

A Japanese man was so enraged by an acquaintance's failure to address him with an honorific that he stabbed the man to death with an umbrella.

Police said the suspect was arrested and confessed to killing a man with the umbrella during a quarrel in the city of Sakuragi.

Honorific terms of address are used constantly in Japan, even among friends, most commonly by adding the suffix "san" to a person's name. Failure to do so is seen as extremely rude.

In recent days another middle-aged man in southwestern Japan was also stabbed to death with an umbrella, this time apparently over who had the right of way on a narrow road.

Prisoner Escapes In Cardboard Box

BERLIN   REUTERS

Police launched a manhunt for a convicted murderer who escaped from prison in a cardboard box.

The 27-year-old Yugoslav outwitted guards by concealing himself in a box he had been given to assemble at the Waldeck prison in eastern Germany.

"He had been working in the prison's box folding department and it appears he got into a box," said a spokesman for the Justice Ministry in the eastern state of Mecklenburg-Vorpommern.

A truck driver unwittingly transported the box out of jail and the prisoner jumped off the vehicle unseen. Police combed the area using helicopters, horses and dogs.

concealed

in a box

Man Tries To Rob Gun Shop With Toy Pistol

PARIS   REUTERS

Armed with a toy pistol, a would-be robber picked himself an unlikely target in central Paris—a gun shop.

Staff at the Armurerie Gare de l'Est in the French capital immediately identified the weapon as harmless. The 26-year-old Mauritanian was subsequently arrested, *Le Parisien* newspaper reported.

SCARECROW GUARDS JAILBIRDS

SAO PAULO | Brazil   REUTERS

A judge on an inspection visit to a Brazilian jail discovered a straw scarecrow dressed in a police uniform on the watchtower "guarding" some 735 jailbirds, police said.

The judge removed the scarecrow, which had apparently been manning the watchtower for days, and took it to the court as evidence. Police opened an investigation.

"It is considered a grave breach of security rules," a police spokesman said. He added that a prison guard should be on the tower at all times in Brazil's prisons, which are plagued with breakouts and riots.

Sniffing Out Shoe Fetish In Man's Attic

TEL AVIV   REUTERS

Israeli police have arrested a computer programmer who got his kicks by stealing and sniffing the shoes and socks of unwitting female colleagues.

Police found 205 pairs of shoes, as well as socks and items of underwear, hidden in the attic of the 33-year-old married man, a spokeswoman for the Sharon region police department said.

"He would take the keys of his co-workers, make copies, and then go to their houses when they weren't home," the spokeswoman said. "We also found ladies underwear, but mainly it was shoes and socks."

The man was caught after 14 women reported missing shoes. A private investigation agency planted one of their own female detectives as a new employee at the high-tech company where the man worked.

The police spokeswoman said that the man became sexually aroused by smelling the shoes and that he swapped stories and shoes over the Internet with others who had the same fetish.

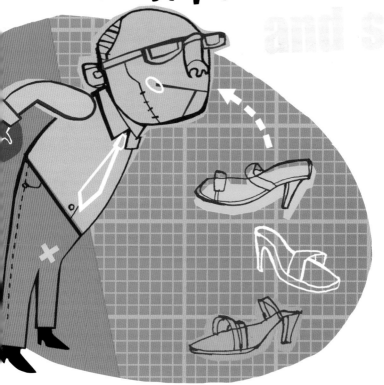

I'd KILL To Win That Election...

MBABANE   REUTERS

Swaziland's ruler warned candidates for October parliamentary elections not to turn to ritual murders for good fortune when campaigning gets under way.

"During election times, we tend to lose our grandmothers, grandfathers and young children. They just disappear. But I want to warn you all that you should not resort to ritual murder," King Mswati III said in a televised address.

Mswati, sub-Saharan Africa's only absolute monarch, dissolved parliament, a day after receiving a draft constitution which maintains a ban on political parties but grants equal rights to women.

Corpses and missing body parts appear occasionally throughout the impoverished southern African kingdom, with at least six cases reported this year alone.

Rituals meant to bring good fortune, often involving the use of human body parts, are still practiced in many parts of Swaziland.

ROBBERS CALL VERY WRONG NUMBER

VANCOUVER | British Columbia   REUTERS

The redial button proved an inconvenient cell-phone feature for three Canadian robbery suspects, providing police with a recording of the crime and an argument over how the loot should be split.

The three men were midway through a hold-up when a cell phone being carried by one of them was jostled and automatically redialed the last number called, police in Burnaby, British Columbia, said.

That number was hooked up to an answering machine whose owner gave a tape of the call to police, said a constable of the Royal Canadian Mounted Police.

On the tape, which was aired on Vancouver-area radio stations, the three could be heard telling the victim "you're being jacked" and later counting more than $100 in cash and arguing about how to divide it.

"YOU'RE BEING JACKED" three Canadian robbery suspects

IT HAS A FAMILIAR RING...

SINGAPORE   REUTERS

An unlucky Singapore thief picked up six years at hard labor after the unique ring of the mobile phone he stole led police straight to him.

Pretending to be a police detective, the man frisked two teenagers in a park, told them to turn their backs and made off with the S$250 ($140) phone, court documents show.

If he had chosen another target in the mobile-mad city state, he might have got off the hook.

His number was up a short while later when the victim heard the characteristic tune he had programmed into the phone. An unsuspecting buyer, who paid $70 in a coffee shop for what he thought was the man's mobile, pointed police to the thief.

For Sale: Car Loaded With Extras—Like Cocaine

BERLIN   REUTERS

German customs unwittingly auctioned a car containing 22 pounds of cocaine, the Customs Investigation Authority (ZFA) in the northern city of Hamburg said.

The Chevrolet was originally imported from Mexico and impounded in 1997 after an X-ray revealed it carried 120 pounds of the drug. But that wasn't all.

"The software used to scan the car in 1997 was not sophisticated enough to pick up the other 10 kilograms," said a Hamburg ZFA spokesman.

The car sat in storage until it was auctioned. The new owner discovered 11 bags of the white powder in the trunk. He returned to customs with the drugs.

HOW'D YOU CATCH ME? WHERE DID I SLIP UP?

RIO DE JANEIRO | Brazil   REUTERS

Crime doesn't pay, especially if a robber demands a ransom be paid to his own bank account.

Police in Rio de Janeiro said such a transaction gave away a Brazilian who, with an accomplice, had stolen a car and a cellular phone at gunpoint.

The desperate owner of the car called the robber on the stolen phone and negotiated the return of his vehicle for a ransom of $345.

The assailant then proceeded to give his personal bank account number for the money to be deposited there. But, after paying the ransom and waiting for the return of the car, it became clear that the robber was not going to give it back.

"Then the owner rushed to us asking for help," an investigator told Reuters. "It was no Swiss account so we quickly found him," he said.

Police tracked the account and seized the suspect over the weekend. He was identified by the van's owner. They also found a stolen car that had been exchanged for the van in his yard.

CRIME DOESN'T PAY

BREAST-TEMPTRESS THIEVES NABBED

BOGOTA | Colombia   REUTERS

Three young Colombian women preyed on men by smearing their breasts with a powerful drug and luring the victims into taking a lick, before making off with their wallets and cars, police said.

The women stood by the side of the road near bars and restaurants in wealthy parts of the capital Bogota, striking seductive poses to lure men driving by to stop, a police spokeswoman told Reuters.

After licking the women's breasts, the men lost all will-power.

They came to their senses hours later to find they had lost their wallets and cars but with no memory of what had happened.

The three women, in their late teens or early 20s, were arrested in Bogota in possession of powerful narcotic pills. "They dissolved the pills in water and rubbed it into their breasts," the spokeswoman said.

Colombia's inventive thieves often dope people to rob them. On rare occasions, these victims have died.

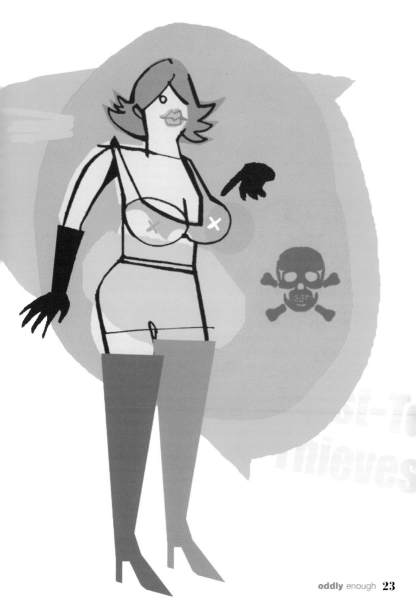

ACCUSED PEEPING TOM GOES HIGH TECH

SAN FRANCISCO REUTERS

Fusing age-old lust with the kind of technology that made Silicon Valley famous, a Californian rigged up a tiny camera on his shoe to look up women's dresses—until he was nabbed by police.

"It's kind of like a modern version of the guy with a mirror on his shoe," a Palo Alto detective said. "It was a pinhole camera—it is something that we use for surveillance purposes."

Police said the man was nabbed at a classic car show when someone noticed that he had little interest in cars and a particular focus on skirted women attending the event.

A camera lens the size of a pinhead was discovered placed on his shoe laces. Police said the man had then linked the lens to a video camera, via a wire threaded up the leg of his pants.

HE WAS NABBED BY POLICE

The Sound Of New Jersey Made Him Snap

GALVESTON | Texas   REUTERS

A Texas jury found a man guilty of aggravated assault for shooting his girlfriend because he thought she was about to say the words "New Jersey."

His attorney unsuccessfully sought his exoneration on grounds that certain words set off an uncontrollable rage in the man, who has a history of mental illness.

Words that triggered a bad reaction in the defendant included "New Jersey," "Wisconsin," "Snickers" and "Mars," the lawyer told the court.

Throughout the three-day trial, the 54-year-old man covered his ears when he thought the words were going to be spoken.

Witnesses used flashcards with the words written out instead of saying them in court.

"When he has one of these episodes, he isn't focused," his lawyer said.

Prosecutors said the man was troubled but not crazy.

He was convicted for shooting his girlfriend three times on March 19, 1999, when he believed she was about to utter the phrase "New Jersey." She survived the attack but died from unrelated causes just before the trial.

In a statement, the man told police: "I had seen that word at my mom's house and then Barbara said what she said (and) I just snapped."

Toddlers Go On Rampage

PARIS   REUTERS

Three-year-old twin boys who disappeared from home then reappeared hours later without their clothes had been off wreaking havoc in a neighbor's empty house, French newspapers reported.

Police initially feared an abduction when the missing boys were discovered late in the evening walking through their home town of Deols, western France, stark naked and holding a bedside lamp.

But a call from a neighbor to report a suspected burglary revealed the boys had broken into a nearby house and gone berserk, emptying out drawers, bouncing on beds, scribbling on walls and gobbling up orange-flavored vitamin pills.

The twins discarded their clothes after getting covered in shampoo and toothpaste during a rampage through the bathroom, squeezing out bottles and tubes.

They grabbed a bedside light and took it away with them thinking it would help them find their way home in the dark.

CHEATING YOUR WAY THROUGH ETHICS

OTTAWA   REUTERS

A group of Canadian engineering students took the art of cheating to its logical conclusion by plagiarizing an essay on ethics, embarrassed academics said.

An associate dean at Ottawa's Carleton University said he would be dealing with 31 students who had been caught submitting essays cribbed from the Internet.

"We're disappointed this has happened in the course on ethics," he told CBC television, noting that those students involved could be suspended or even expelled from the University.

In one case, a student had changed just four words in an essay taken from a Web site, the associate dean added.

cribbed from the Internet

CHANGED JUST FOUR WORDS

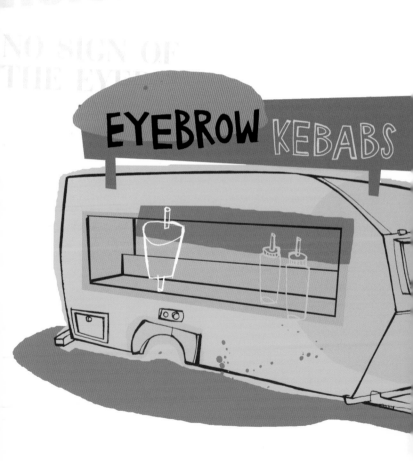

EYEBROW EATEN IN KEBAB VAN ATTACK

LONDON   REUTERS

British police were hunting for a thug who bit off a man's eyebrow and possibly ate it after a drunken fight by a kebab van.

The 34-year-old victim and a friend were set upon as they headed toward the carry-out van in the center of Trowbridge, Wiltshire, in southwest England.

The stocky attacker, in his 30s, launched a violent assault after the victim made an inoffensive comment to two young women, police said.

"He stuck his teeth into the eyebrow and bit it off. It's a possibility that he ate it as shortly afterwards a search was conducted and there was no sign of the eyebrow," a detective constable told Reuters.

World Cup Ultimatum

LONDON   REUTERS

Soccer-mad criminals have been surrendering to British police in the hope of completing a short jail sentence in time to watch the World Cup, British newspapers reported.

In "Operation Red Card," police in Hertfordshire, north of London, sent a simple message to defendants who had been failing to turn up in court: surrender now or spend the World Cup in a police cell with no television, according to the *Evening Standard* newspaper.

"One man even turned up to court with his bag packed, expecting a short spell in prison," it quoted Hertfordshire's Sergeant Nigel Eastaugh as saying.

"No doubt he wanted to get his sentence over and done with to make sure he would be free again in time for the World Cup," Sergeant Eastaugh added.

The paper said the 296 letters sent to offenders' last known addresses had resulted in 17 people walking into local police stations to face charges such as assault and theft.

Ten had turned up for court hearings, the paper said.

Soccer-mad criminals

knife-wielding

REST IN PEACE, DUDE

BRASILIA | Brazil   REUTERS

Brazilian police have seized two bogus funerary agents who transported a big batch of marijuana in a hearse, complete with a coffin, from the border town of Foz do Iguacu to the capital Brasilia.

A federal police spokesman said police found 198 pounds of the drug that the suspects—a man and a woman—were loading into the false bottom of the hearse under the coffin during a stopover.

"That is a significant amount of weed, but what makes it unusual is, of course, the coffin, which also had traces of the drug," a spokesman told Reuters.

Police said they had evidence the couple had been running the self-styled funerary service for several months. The alleged traffickers may get between three and 15 years in jail if convicted.

ROBBERS SORRY, BUT...

MANILA   REUTERS

Two men apologized to a Philippine taxi driver for having to rob him, but their goodwill was brief when they stabbed him six times for not giving them enough loot.

Police said the driver was in the hospital but out of danger after the robbery in Manila.

"We're very sorry, sir. But we need your money," he said the robbers told him.

He gave the knife-wielding robbers his day's earnings of 500 pesos ($9.43) and a diver's watch, saying that was all he had.

"You're a liar," police said one of the suspects responded before stabbing him.

WOULD-BE ROBBER GETS NO RESPECT

LITTLE ROCK REUTERS

A would-be bank robber couldn't get any respect, police said.

The 23-year-old robber entered a bank and told a teller to stuff a bag full of money. His other hand was allegedly thrust in his pocket to make it seem like he was carrying a gun, police said.

The first teller laughed at the robbery attempt and told him the bank was out of money. The robber then went to another teller a few feet away and tried the same method to rob the bank, police said.

This time, he was handed deposit slips as the teller told him that if he wanted to steal money, he had better first put some money in the bank.

The tellers told police the man then threw down his plastic bag in disgust and walked out of the bank. He was arrested a few minutes later about four blocks away after bank employees called police for help.

EMPLOYEES CALLED POLICE FOR HELP

arrested a few minutes later

Man Holds Up Gas Station To Pay Taxi Fare

DORTMUND | Germany   REUTERS

A German robber short of cash during a taxi ride held up a gas station to pay his unwitting driver, police said.

The man asked the driver to stop outside the gas station, robbed the cashier at gunpoint and returned to the waiting taxi with several hundred euros (dollars), a police spokesman said.

The driver knew nothing of the crime and helped his well-dressed customer make a clean getaway.

"He had no problem paying the driver since he had plenty of money for the fare," said a police spokesman.

ELDERLY VIAGRA THIEF STRIKES AGAIN

MARSEILLE | France   REUTERS

An elderly man has robbed a pharmacy in the southern French city of Marseille for the fourth time in less than a year, each time making off with its full stock of the anti-impotence drug Viagra.

Each time he strikes, he appears at closing time armed with a knife and marches the three female members of staff to the cupboard where they keep the coveted blue pills, Marseille police said.

He then leaves quietly with his stash and the day's takings.

Police said they did not know whether the thief was stealing the Viagra for his personal use, or to resell the pills illegally with a hefty premium.

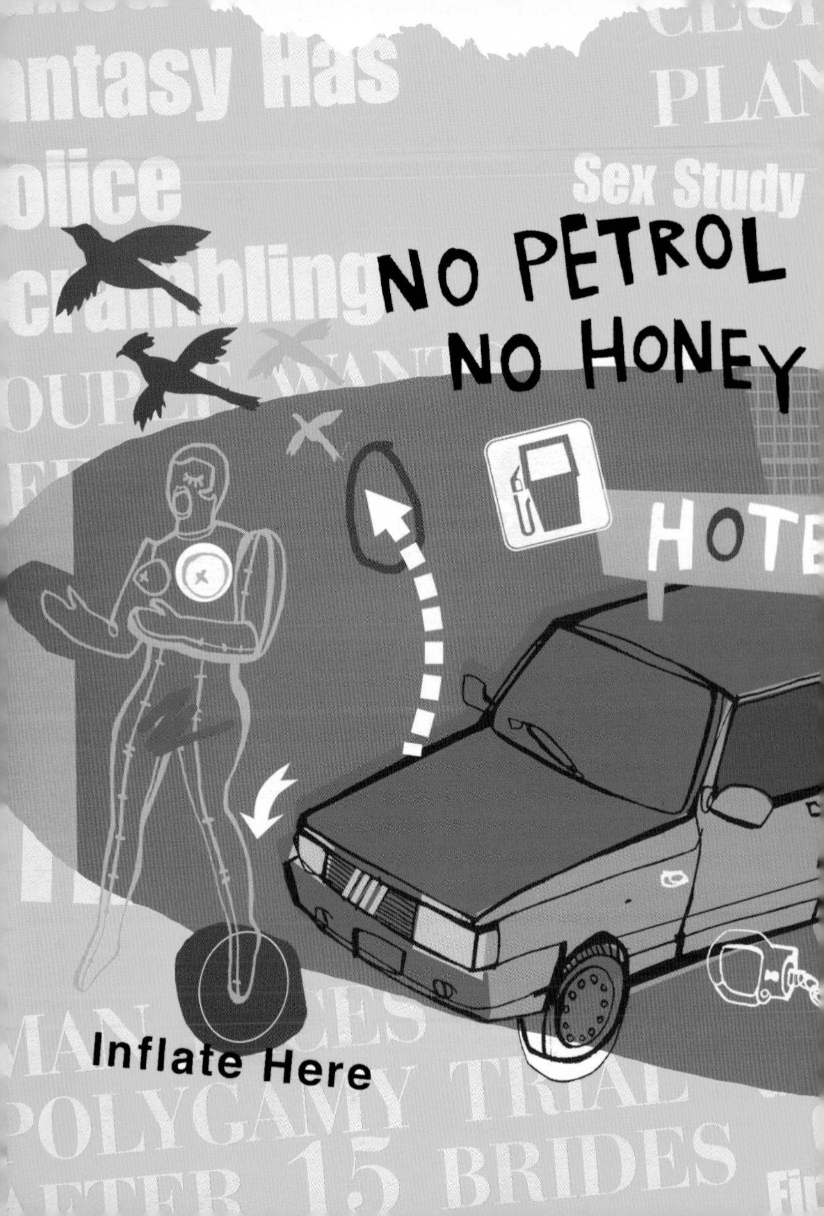

ntasy Has
PLAN
olice
Sex Study
crambling
NO PETROL
NO HONEY
HOTE
Inflate Here
POLYGAMY TRIAL
AFTER 15 BRIDES

CHAPTER 2

Sex, Love And Marriage

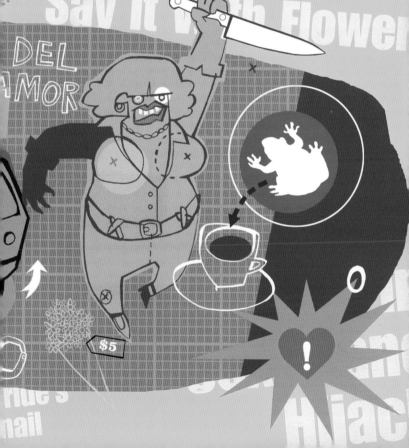

Naked Kidnap Fantasy Has Police Scrambling

EDMONTON | Alberta

REUTERS

Canadian police in a frantic search for an abducted woman dispatched a SWAT team to her home before officers on a routine patrol across town found her naked and bound in the back of a car.

But police in Edmonton, Alberta, soon realized they had a problem—she did not want to be rescued.

It emerged that the 17-year-old female and a man at the scene were engaged in a role-playing game, but not before the man was arrested and the woman sent to hospital for examination. She was less than co-operative, police said.

"She did answer questions, but she wasn't very forthcoming with the detectives. They pieced it together that it was some form of fantasy scenario on the part of the people involved," an Edmonton police spokesman said.

"It wasn't so funny for us because we burned up a lot of taxpayers' money dealing with this."

The saga began when a man called 911 to report that he had been talking on the phone to the woman. He said that during their call, the woman had said someone had broken into her house. The line then went dead.

Phone Sex Operator Gets Masturbation Settlement

MIAMI REUTERS

A Florida phone sex operator has won a workers' compensation settlement claiming she was injured after regularly masturbating at work, her lawyer said.

The lawyer told Reuters he was not sure whether the Fort Lauderdale woman's claim was the first of its kind, but it certainly was out of the ordinary.

He said his client agreed to a "minimal settlement" earlier this month. He declined to disclose the amount.

During the course of her claim for workers' compensation benefits, the now 40-year-old employee of Fort Lauderdale's CFP Enterprises Inc. said she developed carpal tunnel syndrome—also known as repetitive motion injury—in both hands from masturbating as many as seven times a day while speaking with callers, said the attorney, who spoke about the case this week on the condition that his client's name not be revealed.

"She was told to do whatever it takes to keep the person on the phone as long as possible," he said.

The woman used one hand to answer the telephone and the other to note customers' names and fetishes and to give herself an orgasm during the verbal exchanges.

Groom Chokes On Bride's Fingernail

TEHRAN   REUTERS

An Iranian bridegroom, following local custom by licking honey from his bride's finger during their marriage ceremony, choked to death on one of her false nails.

The *Jam-e Jam* newspaper said the 28-year-old groom died on the spot in the northwestern city of Qazvin while the bride was rushed to a hospital after fainting from shock.

Iranian couples lick honey from each other's fingers when they get married so that their life together starts sweetly.

A FULL-SERVICE FILL-UP

SHANGHAI   REUTERS

Enterprising gas stations in western China have taken service to new heights by offering sex with a tank of gasoline.

Some of the more than 1,000 filling stations in the region of Ningxia have been luring motorists with the services of a prostitute along with gas and diesel oil, an industry publication said.

"Sometimes there is no clear dividing line whether the customers come for gas or sex, but the sex service is based on the condition that you have to buy petrol first," said a publication of the official Xinhua news agency.

"The term 'no money, no honey' has changed into 'no petrol, no honey'," it said.

bride rushed to hospital

AGING PLAYBOY OFFERS JACKPOT TO FINAL BEDMATE

BERLIN REUTERS

An aging Berlin playboy has come up with an unusual offer to lure women into his bed by promising the last woman he sleeps with an inheritance of about $244,000.

The 72-year-old disco owner, well-known for his numerous sex partners, said he could imagine no better way to die than in the arms of an attractive young woman—preferably under 30.

"I put it all in my last will and testament—the last woman who sleeps with me gets all the money," the man told *Bild* newspaper.

"I want to pass away in the most beautiful moment of my life. First a lot of fun with a beautiful woman, then wild sex, a final orgasm—and it will all end with a heart attack and then I'm gone."

The man said "applicants" shouldn't wait long because of his advanced age.

"It could end very soon," he said. "Maybe even tomorrow."

72-year-old disco owner

Say It With Flowers?

PETALUMA | Calif   REUTERS

He said it with flowers. She answered with a knife in the back.

A Petaluma, California, woman has been sentenced to six months in jail for stabbing her husband with a 13-inch knife after he brought home two bunches of flowers for her, the *Santa Rosa Press Democrat* reported.

"She didn't think he should have spent that kind of money on flowers," the prosecutor told the newspaper.

The 33-year-old husband, whose name was not released, drove himself to a nearby hospital where he was given four stitches and then released, the newspaper said.

The 28-year-old wife was initially charged with assault with a deadly weapon and spousal abuse, but these charges were dropped when she agreed to plead no contest to felony battery with serious bodily injury.

deadly
weapon

Wife Risks Jail For Reading Husband's Mail

ROME REUTERS

Curiosity killed the cat and it could land one Italian wife in jail for a year.

A man in the northeastern city of Turin has taken his wife to court for repeatedly opening his personal mail, despite his stream of pleas to stop.

The Italian news agency ANSA said a Turin court had opened an inquiry into the complaint.

ANSA did not name the couple but said the wife's prying could be punished by a prison sentence or a 516 euro (dollar) fine.

DUMPED LOVER UNCAGES BOYFRIEND'S BIRDS

BRUSSELS REUTERS

A woman dumped by her bird-loving boyfriend took her revenge by setting free some 350 of his feathered friends, a Belgian paper said.

The unidentified woman opened the doors of three aviaries in the Belgian coastal town of Bredene, letting fly hundreds of her ex's birds, most of them canaries, *Het Volk* daily said.

Neighbors and friends of the boyfriend had since helped catch about 100 of them, it said.

"We've been catching birds for the past three days," a town local told the daily. "The animals are so tame you can catch them with a fishnet.

"It's incredible that someone would let those birds free out of revenge," he added.

Addicts: The Ultimate Drug Test Kits

NEW DELHI REUTERS

Indian police have found something more reliable than sniffer dogs or imported testing kits when they need to quickly verify their latest drug haul is the real thing—junkies.

Drugs sold on the streets of New Delhi, such as smack (also known as brown sugar), hash and heroin are often so heavily mixed with anything from boot polish to household dust that police have no idea what they have, the *Hindustan Times* newspaper reported.

So they call on addicts, going to particular slums for different drugs and paying their "tasters" a fee.

"While drugs like opium and hash are easily detected by their smell, we generally get stuck with brown sugar and heroin seizures," the *Times* quoted one officer saying.

"In fact, sometimes even the imported testing kits give arbitrary results if the heroin is not of fine quality. That is when we call in the tasters. And they are never wrong."

IMPORTED
TESTING KITS

"Corpse" Turns Out To Be Sex Doll

MUNICH | Germany   REUTERS

A Munich man suspected of murder after he was seen carrying what a neighbor thought was a body into his flat has cleared his name by showing police his collection of rubber sex dolls.

A police spokeswoman said the neighbor called to say he saw the man carrying a "corpse" into the apartment. Police responding to the call found the suspect to be "surprised and disturbed" by their questions at first.

Told they were investigating a murder, he showed them the dolls.

INTERRUPTED SEX CLAIM

BERLIN   REUTERS

A German couple is demanding compensation from a tour operator because a maid repeatedly interrupted them while they were having sex in their hotel room during a holiday in Cuba, a court spokesman said.

The man and wife filed a lawsuit at a district court in Hanover seeking a refund because they said the maid walked in on two occasions during intercourse even though they had a "Do Not Disturb" sign outside the door.

They are seeking about $4,000 in damages from the holiday company. But the company said the hotel's failings only amounted to an "inconvenience" and did not warrant such high compensation.

MILE HIGH CLUB FORCES PLANE REFIT?

LONDON REUTERS

Virgin Atlantic Airways is to replace tables in its newest planes because passengers have broken them during illicit trysts, the *Sun* newspaper said.

The $200 million Airbus A340-600 has a "mother and baby room" with a plastic table meant for changing diapers. But passengers have destroyed them by using them for sex.

"Those determined to join the Mile High Club will do so despite the lack of comforts," a Virgin spokeswoman was quoted as saying.

"We don't mind couples having a good time, but this is not something that we would encourage because of air regulations."

Sex Study Dents Image Of Latin Lover

MADRID REUTERS

A survey of Spaniards' sexual habits has dented the image of the spontaneous Latin lover by showing that 77 percent plan in advance when they will have sex.

The survey by the Spanish Federation of Sexology Societies (FESS), based on telephone interviews with more than 1,200 people, showed that 18- to 24-year-olds were most likely to plan the day and place newspapers reported.

"The Iberian macho is a myth now, but we have gained in tenderness and communication," a sexologist was quoted as saying by *El Mundo*.

women know what
they want

SEX TOYS FOR WOM

Handcuffs: The New Must-Have For Sexy Women

BERLIN   REUTERS

Handcuffs are the fastest-selling item at five new shops tailored for women by Germany's biggest retailer of sex merchandise, the store chain said.

Beate Uhse AG said handcuffs have been flying off the shelves of stores it opened this year to focus on sex toys for women rather than the traditional male clientele.

"Women's sexual appetites are steeped more in the realm of fantasy—they like to use their imagination more than men," said a spokeswoman for Beate Uhse at corporate headquarters in Flensburg.

"The shop had just opened and the handcuffs were all gone the first day," she said.

Beate Uhse AG's five recently opened shops reported that an 90 percent of their customers have been women.

"This just goes to show that these days women know what they want and they're not shy about getting it," the spokeswoman added.

Couple Divorced Over Frog In Teacup

LUSAKA   REUTERS

A Zambian man divorced his wife after he found a frog in a cup of tea she gave him, a Lusaka newspaper reported.

"One time I found a frog in a cup of tea she had served me. That is the reason I went for another woman," the independent newspaper quoted the husband as telling a community court.

The court granted him a divorce, saying it was clear from the evidence presented that the couple's marriage could not be saved.

MAN DIVORCES QUARRELSOME WIFE FOR MUTE WOMAN

SANAA   REUTERS

A Yemeni man divorced his first wife because she was loud and argumentative and picked a deaf and mute woman as his new bride, a local newspaper said.

Al-Thawra daily said a 40-year-old man from the southern Dhamar province became so tired of his wife's "screaming and endless disputes" that he left her after 15 years to remarry.

"He chose one deprived of hearing and speech and who is quiet and mild-mannered," it said.

COUPLE DIES IN SEX-PLANE HIJACK

MIAMI REUTERS

An elderly couple who chartered a small plane on the pretext of having sex in the sky died when the plane plunged into the sea off the Florida Keys after they tried to hijack it to Cuba, U.S. authorities said.

The unidentified couple scuffled with the pilot when the Piper Cherokee was about 40 miles south of Key West, sending the small plane plunging into deep water in the Florida Straits.

The 36-year-old pilot managed to scramble out of the sinking plane and suffered only cuts and bruises. But the man and woman apparently were trapped.

"This is what the pilot is telling us," an FBI agent said. "An elderly Cuban couple in their 60s asked to be taken on a 'Mile High' tour. Once they were up in the air ... they demanded to be taken to Cuba.

"There was a scuffle and the pilot tried to maneuver the plane. The man fell on the throttle and made it so that he (the pilot) couldn't fly the plane. He had to ditch the plane."

Local media said the pilot was the co-owner of a tour company called Fly Key West, which on its Web site advertises "Mile High Club" tours for people who want to have sex in a plane.

"Come fly the very friendly skies," the Web site beckons. "Cleaner than a hotel room. Brand new Key West Mile High Club souvenir sheets on every flight."

The company offers a "Quickie" flight of 35 minutes for $199, up to a 55-minute sunset tour for $349.

NO LONGER
SATISFIED HER
SEXUALLY

Public Humiliation Perfectly Normal, Court Rules

ROME   REUTERS

Does your wife make your life hell, humiliating you in front of friends and family, insulting you day after day and even berating you for not giving her pleasure in bed?

Italy's highest court has ruled that this is not exceptional, and if you divorce your wife you must still pay her alimony, according to a report in the daily *Il Messaggero*.

The Court of Cassation has ruled that a Naples magistrate who left his wife after 10 years of such treatment was nevertheless at fault for ending

the marriage and should pay up, the paper said.

"That woman massacred me for 10 years," the man said after the ruling. His ex-wife argued that her behavior was normal in a married couple and she could not be blamed for a few "outbursts." The court agreed, but the ex-husband was seething.

"Not a day went by without her humiliating me in front of everybody. She would even scream at me that I no longer satisfied her sexually. And now I have to support her?"

MAN FACES POLYGAMY TRIAL AFTER 15 BRIDES

MANAGUA | Nicaragua   REUTERS

A Nicaraguan man caught trying to sign up for what authorities say was his 15th bride in the Managua municipal registry is facing trial for polygamy, officials said.

Registry records show the man, 38, married 14 times between 1998 and 2000, a registrar said.

The man, a former civil servant who now works as a trucker, is under house arrest facing trial in a week's time on charges of "illegally contracting marriage."

He told local newspapers, "It's normal to be a womanizer" but said he only married once after divorcing his first wife.

Authorities discovered the alleged multiple marriages when the man supposedly tried to register his most recent bride. It apears that previous marriage registrations had all passed through unnoticed at first because the marriage registry had only been computerized in 2001.

"It's normal to be a womanizer"

Parking Lots of Love

ROME   REUTERS

All roads lead to Rome, but amorous young Italians anxious to escape mama's beady eye might be tempted to take a detour to the country's first "Love Car Park."

The Tuscan town of Vinci, more commonly known for its Renaissance artist son Leonardo, is renovating a car park complete with soft lighting and special trash bins for condoms.

"We're just recognizing that young people love each other," Mayor Giancarlo Faenzi told Reuters by telephone.

"If you don't face that fact, you're simply closing your eyes to reality and you just end up sending them a kilometer down the road," he said, adding that the town was still deciding whether to install a condom machine.

The back seat often acts as a substitute bed for those Italians who live with their parents well into their 30s.

Even Prime Minister Silvio Berlusconi famously reminisced about how "many of us first kissed our girl in a Fiat 500."

Italians talk of a "Car-ma Sutra," illustrating positions best suited to specific car models, though no one can ever remember the name of the book.

Car sex is not illegal in strongly Catholic Italy—as long as the windows are covered up.

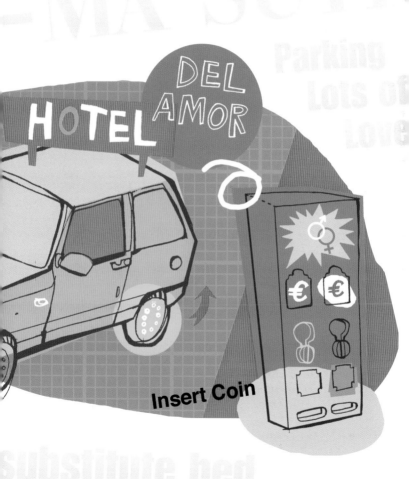

Sorry For Sex In The Sand

PAINESVILLE | Ohio   REUTERS

A couple who had sex on a popular lakeside beach in Ohio were ordered by a judge to apologize to shocked beachgoers in newspaper advertisements, or go to jail.

A Painesville judge ordered the couple to run ads in two local newspapers apologizing for their public display of ardor at Mentor Headlands State Park Beach on Lake Erie near Cleveland.

The judge, who is known for his innovative sentences, gave them the choice of complying with his order or going to jail for 22 days for public indecency.

The couple, who engaged in oral sex, agreed to complete two days of community service and submit the ads, which will be worded, "I apologize for any activities that I engaged in that were offensive and disrespectful."

Several families at the beach complained to lifeguards after seeing the couple's tryst.

PUPPY LOVE... GIRL WEDS DOG TO WARD OFF EVIL

NEW DELHI | India   REUTERS

A nine-year-old Indian girl was married to a dog amid religious chants after a priest told her parents the wedding would ward off evil, a government official said.

The marriage between the girl and a mongrel dog called "Bachchan" took place in Khannan village, some 35 miles northwest of Calcutta.

"The priest told the girl's family, who are poor tribal farmers, that because new teeth appeared on her upper gums rather than her lower gums, it was a bad omen and she would die," a government welfare officer told Reuters by phone.

"The priest said to ward off danger to her life, the parents should marry the girl to a dog, which they did," he added.

Officials and witnesses said the girl married the dog, which has a brown, white and black coat, on a raised dais amid chanting of religious hymns and the feeding of the canine "groom" with rice.

The communist government in West Bengal said it planned to investigate the wedding, although it was merely a ceremonial one and the girl would be free to marry a man when she was older.

MAN CUTS OFF PENIS, TOSSES IT TO HIS WIFE

MANILA   REUTERS

A Filipino man cut off his penis and tossed it through a window to his estranged wife in a bid to prove his fidelity.

The man wrapped the severed member in a newspaper and threw it through the window of his wife's parents' house in the northwestern town of Malasiqui, the *Philippine Star* said.

"So you will not suspect I am courting another girl," the *Star* said the man shouted before he hobbled off into the night.

His shocked wife gave the severed penis straight to police, who then sought the help of an embalmer to preserve it until her husband could be found, the Philippine paper said.

Heartbroken By Divorce, Man Burns Family Assets

STOCKHOLM   REUTERS

A Swedish man, desolate after his wife filed for divorce, converted the family's shares and mutual funds into cash and burned the money— 700,000 crowns ($81,300) in banknotes, a newspaper reported.

"Bitterness is not uncommon in connection with divorces but it is almost unique that one of the spouses puts fire to all their wealth," the public prosecutor in the town of Jonkoping in southern Sweden said during an interview with the daily *Aftonbladet* newspaper.

WHIPS AND CHAINS GROUNDS FOR DIVORCE

ROME REUTERS

It might have seemed like a bit of slap and tickle at the time, but an Italian court has ruled that sadomasochism is justifiable grounds for divorce.

Italy's highest appeals court has backed a woman's claim that her ex-husband was responsible for the break-up of their marriage after making excessive demands for sadomasochistic sex, leaving her psychologically and physically bruised.

The decision overturned a lower court ruling which had said the wealthy couple were equally responsible for the divorce since, while she had to put up with his sexual predilections, he had to suffer her arguing and plate throwing.

After hearing evidence from psychoanalysts who treated the woman for a nervous breakdown during the marriage, the higher court ruled the man should have been more sympathetic to his wife and not insisted that she join in his sexual games.

wrapped the
severed member
in a newspaper

MOANING TOO LOUD— SWINGERS' CLUB SHUTS

BERLIN   REUTERS

A swingers' club in Berlin has been forced to shut because a court ruled that members' moans and shrieks of pleasure broke noise regulations.

Partner-swapping customers at the ground-floor club called "Zwielicht"—a German word meaning both "twilight" and "dubious"—upset those living upstairs, a Berlin court ruled this week.

"There are other clubs and brothels in this area and the customers there don't make so much noise. They are more discreet," a court spokeswoman said.

A Berlin actress, who lives above the club, told the court she was tired of seeing men wearing only bathrobes getting out of limousines on their way into the club.

See The Sights, Starting With These Two Here...

BARE BREASTED STRIPPER

BERLIN   REUTERS

A tour bus filled with beer-drinking passengers and a handful of bare-breasted strippers is plying the night-time streets of Berlin, giving the German capital a hot new tourist attraction.

The double-decker bus cruises past the city's main tourist spots, including the Brandenburg Gate, the Reichstag parliament building, the chancellery, the state opera house, Tiergarten park and the Victory Column on a three-hour tour.

But the crowd on board seems less interested in Berlin's cultural offerings than it is in the tour guide, who slowly disrobes during her commentary, and her two "assistants" who keep spirits high with a series of strip shows.

"It's a terrific way to see Berlin, but the windows are a bit too steamed up to see much outside," said a construction worker called Sascha, cooling off with a beer after a stripper named Jenny, 20, rested on his leg.

It's a terrific way to see Berlin

Near-Naked Women Won't Be Drafted

BOGOTA | Colombia REUTERS

Busty, bikini-clad models won't be air-dropped into Colombia's combat zones after all.

The war-torn Andean nation's first female defense minister, Marta Lucia Ramirez, canceled the army's campaign to seduce Marxist rebel defectors with pictures of near-naked women.

In the thousands of pocket-sized portraits already printed, and waiting to be air-dropped over battlefields, the voluptuous vixens were presented as a perk for desertion.

"Desert! And obtain benefits," read one pamphlet, depicting a brunette stretching provocatively in a striped bikini.

An army officer, who declined to be identified, said the portraits were taken from an Internet porn site.

Ramirez told local press the posters did not fit within the government's concept of "rehabilitating these boys, re-socializing them and making them useful to society."

Of Colombia's more than 20,000 Marxist rebels, about 70 percent are men—stacking the odds against the male fighters, many of whom are still in their teens.

To have sexual relations with female rebels, male guerrillas must first ask permission from higher-ranking officers.

CALL FOR CONDOM TESTERS SWAMPED BY OFFERS

LONDON   REUTERS

An appeal for British students to volunteer to rigorously road-test condoms and be paid 100 pounds ($158) has been overwhelmed by applicants, manufacturer Condomi said.

Within a week of the appeal for sexually active men and women to come forward, the firm had received 10,000 applications and is combing the list selecting 100 who will get lucky.

The winners will be required to perform what the firm called "rigorous pleasure tests" on its entire range and fill in a detailed questionnaire on their reactions.

"The response has been phenomenal," the marketing manager said. "It is quite surprising how much detail some people go into when answering intimate questions."

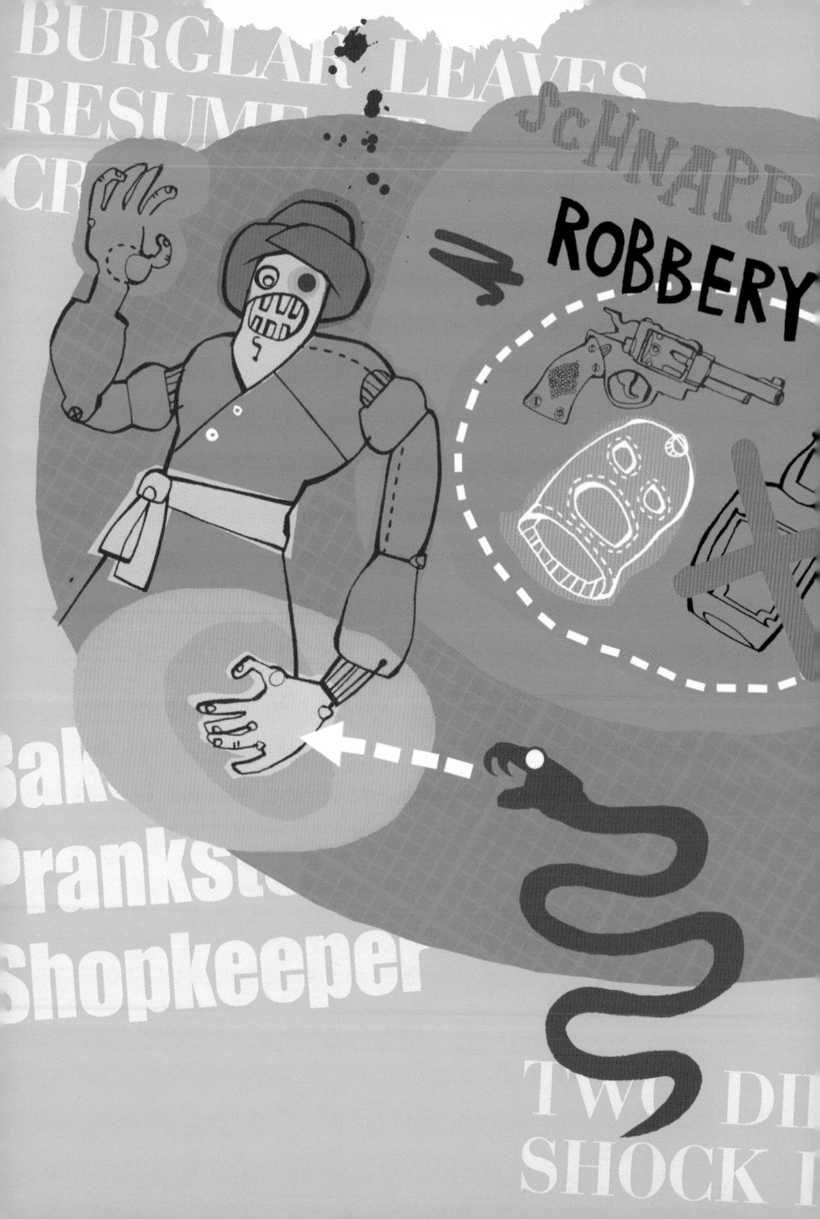
BURGLAR LEAVES
RESUME
ROBBERY
Shopkeeper
SHOCK

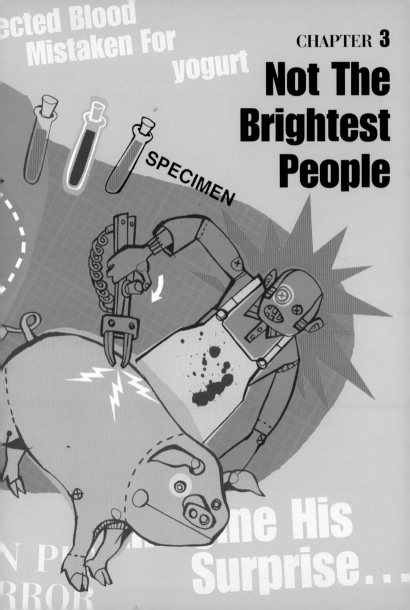

Baked Bean Foot Prankster Dupes Shopkeeper

LONDON   REUTERS

A young shop assistant was tricked into letting a complete stranger smear her bare feet with baked beans and syrup "for charity."

The woman in her 20s was alone in the Edinburgh shop when the man came in, police said.

She agreed to his bizarre request, which he said was aimed at raising money for a charity.

"He brought foodstuffs with him and made her lie back with her eyes closed before proceeding to pour gunk on her feet. He then asked her if she could identify what they were," said a police spokeswoman.

The stranger, believed to be in his early 30s, also took several photographs, particularly of her feet.

Lothian and Borders Police said the man then thanked the woman and left. It was only when she told her roommates about it later that she became alarmed.

TWO DIE IN PIG SHOCK HORROR

BUDAPEST   REUTERS

The annual pre-Christmas swine slaughter in a southwestern Hungarian village came to a shocking end after one man died of electrocution while trying to stun a pig, whose owner then died of a heart attack.

Celebrations at the pig-killing party in Darvaspuszta took a turn for the worse when a visiting Croatian man shocked himself to death while trying to knock out a pig with a homemade electric pig stunner, national news agency MTI said.

A local man ended up in the hospital with an irregular heart rhythm after attempting a rescue by trying to unplug the device.

The accident so upset the pig's owner he suffered a heart attack and died.

There was no word on the fate of the pig.

Infected Blood Mistaken For Yogurt

RIO DE JANEIRO   REUTERS

Two Brazilian car thieves may have drunk vials of HIV-infected blood—thinking it was a yogurt drink—found in a stolen car, officials said.

Over the New Year's weekend, six armed bandits overpowered a worker at a medical laboratory in the remote western state of Rondonia and stole his car while he was on the way to the airport to ship blood samples to a distant laboratory, a security spokesman told Reuters.

"The blood samples came from AIDS patients and were being shipped for further tests," the spokesman said.

The thieves sped out of town, but made a brief stop at a bar on their way. After a few stiff drinks, two members of the gang uncovered the vials and gulped them down, mistaking them for drinkable yogurt, the spokesman added.

"I don't know how it happened, but the culprits told reporters here that they were drunk and confused and didn't know what they were doing," the spokesman said.

Police caught four of the alleged robbers some 50 miles down the road after the car broke down.

drunk and
confused

BURGLAR LEAVES RESUMÉ AT CRIME SCENE

ZURICH   REUTERS

Famous criminals have been known to leave calling cards, but one burglar in Switzerland went a step further, accidentally leaving his resumé behind after a break-in.

"His name and address were written on it and so we paid him a little visit," a spokesman for the canton of Basel police force said. "I assume he realized at some point that he had lost something and so I don't suppose he was very surprised."

Police said the 19-year-old Hungarian was arrested on suspicion of burglary in Oberwil, near the French border, and stealing camera equipment valued at 10,000 Swiss francs ($6,720).

Snake Charmer Not Charming Enough

KUALA LUMPUR   REUTERS

A Malaysian snake charmer who apparently lost patience with his lazy cobra was killed after he pulled the snake out of its box and was bitten, a newspaper reported.

The 23-year-old victim died on the Indonesian island of Batam, where he was performing at a fair, the *New Sunday Times* reported.

A fellow performer said the victim, having difficulty getting his snake to come out of its box, pulled it out and placed it on the floor.

"However, without warning, the snake bit his left hand," he added.

The victim died a few hours later.

Man Shoots Six At His Birthday Party

OSLO   REUTERS

A Norwegian accidentally shot and wounded six of his friends at a surprise party to celebrate his 40th birthday, police said.

The man, who found out the surprise party was to take place in a forest cabin in south Norway, hid behind trees near the cabin with a shotgun. As about 30 guests began to arrive, the man planned to turn the surprise on his friends.

He blasted off one round in the air

meaning it as a joke to shock the partygoers. But when he came out from his hiding place, he tripped and the gun went off again, badly hurting one woman in the legs and slightly injuring five others.

"Seven people were taken to hospital in Fredrikstad including the man who shot. He wasn't physically hurt but in deep shock," a police spokesman said.

The party was canceled.

SO, WAIT—I DON'T GET THE JOB?

OKLAHOMA CITY   REUTERS

Your employment interview probably isn't going well when your prospective boss calls the police in to arrest you.

A 20-year-old applicant was hauled away from an interview for a job with a construction company in Stillwater, Oklahoma, after employees recognized the job applicant as the person seen on a surveillance videotape robbing the same business just one day before, police said.

"When he went out there to apply for the job, there was no one there. So he just helped himself to some items and left," police said. "However, he was caught on videotape."

A day after the robbery, the man applied for a job with the construction company and was arrested.

He didn't get the job.

HE GOES, AND SO DOES HIS CAR

BERLIN   REUTERS

A German driver who got out of his car on a hill to relieve himself found his car at the bottom of a river after he forgot to apply the hand brake, police said.

"At first he tried to claim his car was stolen but the police immediately found this wasn't the case," said a police spokeswoman in the eastern German city of Leipzig.

When the salvage team arrived the next morning, the car was irreparable. "He can expect a fine for parking on the sidewalk and not securing the car properly," the spokesman said.

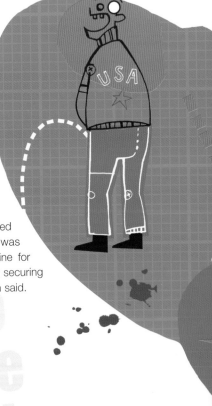

forgot to apply the handbrake

Imagine His Surprise...

TEHRAN   REUTERS

Iranian police are looking for a phony sorcerer who conned a man into believing he was invisible and could rob banks, the *Jam-e Jam* newspaper said.

Customers at a Tehran bank quickly overpowered the deluded robber after he started snatching banknotes from their hands.

Appearing in court, the repentant thief said he paid five million rials ($625) to a man who gave him some spells and told him to tie them to his arm to become invisible.

"I made a mistake. I understand now what a big trick was played on me," the would-be bank robber was reported as telling the judge.

PHONY SORCERE

SUSPICIOUS

NEIGHBOR

SMOOTH TALKING CRIMINAL FOOLS POLICE

LONDON　　REUTERS

Red-faced British police promised to find out why officers allowed a burglar to walk free after they accepted his made-up story over the telephone.

Newspapers reported that the mix-up started when a suspicious neighbor called police in Manchester after he saw a man loitering near a friend's van.

Instead of sending out a patrol car, officers asked that the suspect be put on the telephone—and then accepted his story that he was not committing a crime.

Police later admitted the smooth-talking criminal made off with tools from the van valued at £600 ($1,000).

"It is extremely embarrassing ... I was appalled by the story," a Manchester police spokesman told BBC radio.

"I'm determined we will put this right and mount a full investigation to find out what went wrong," he said.

The police spokesman said the force was overstretched on the night of the embarrassing crime but was "determined to catch the perpetrator."

"IT'S EXTREMELY EMBARRASSING..."

They Don't Teach This In Driver's Ed

BERLIN REUTERS

A German couple stunned highway police when they were spotted changing places behind the wheel while driving at 50 miles per hour, police said.

"It's not a trick I would recommend," said a police spokeswoman.

Police found the Mercedes contained a sleeping baby and some hashish, the spokeswoman said. The 25-year-old male driver had no driver's license.

The couple, stopped in central Germany, was briefly detained and fined but allowed to continue the journey.

POSTER BOY FOR BAD DRIVING

LONDON REUTERS

A one-armed drunk driver clutching his mobile phone to his ear as he sped down a city street and jumped a red light has been fined and banned from driving for 18 months.

The motorist, who lost half of his right arm in an accident, was found to be well over the legal alcohol limit when stopped by police in Swansea.

"I think it would be fair to say this is a pretty unusual case," the superintendent of South Wales police force told Reuters.

"Using a mobile phone while driving, driving over the limit and going through a red light are all concerns in their own right. We urge the public not to do any of these things in isolation, let alone all together," he added.

You Are The Weakest Link...

BERLIN   REUTERS

A German bank robber who forgot to cut open eye slits in his mask and lifted it up to demand money was convicted and sentenced to four years in jail, prosecutors said.

The robber, dubbed "Germany's dumbest criminal" by *Bild* newspaper, had entered a bank in a western town with a burlap bag over his head. Bumping into bank customers on his way to the teller, he pulled out a plastic knife and a toy pistol.

He then lifted the front of his mask to look at the teller and demand money. The robber was told the safe couldn't be opened and he fled. But he was easily identified from the security cameras behind the teller and soon arrested.

"He was a real amateur," said Giessen police spokesman Gerald Frost. "He lifted the mask and looked straight into the camera. He was quickly identified and arrested a day later."

TOOTHY EVIDENCE CONVICTS "BUMBLING ROBBER"

MIAMI   REUTERS

A man the FBI dubbed the "bumbling bank robber" was convicted after investigators matched his DNA to the gold teeth knocked out when a van hit the fleeing suspect, prosecutors said.

The man was convicted of bank robbery in U.S. District Court.

On Sept. 30, 2002, he walked into a Wachovia Bank in Miami, pulled a gun from his pocket and robbed a teller of about $16,000, according to trial evidence. As he ran out of the bank, he stuffed the gun into his waistband, accidentally firing it into his pants. The bullet missed him but when he stepped into the street he was hit by a van delivering school lunches in the area, investigators said.

The robber managed to stumble to a waiting car, leaving two gold teeth, his gun and hat lying in the street, prosecutors said. The FBI later matched DNA from the teeth with his DNA, proving he had been in the bank.

He was arrested a few days after the robbery at a Miami hotel he'd booked into, where agents found a sock full of money from the robbery stuffed into his trousers.

firing it into his pants

IF YOU DRINK, DON'T ROB

GRAZ | Austria   REUTERS

A man went to rob a bank in the Austrian city of Graz but was found by police asleep in his car after downing a bottle of schnapps for courage, police said.

A passer-by alerted the police after noticing that the parked car had different number plates at the front and back, a police spokesman told Reuters.

On the seat next to the slumbering driver police found a balaclava, a pistol and an empty bottle of high-proof schnapps.

The 33-year-old man admitted he had planned to rob the bank but had drunk the schnapps to calm his nerves. He was arrested for questioning and will have to answer charges of attempted robbery.

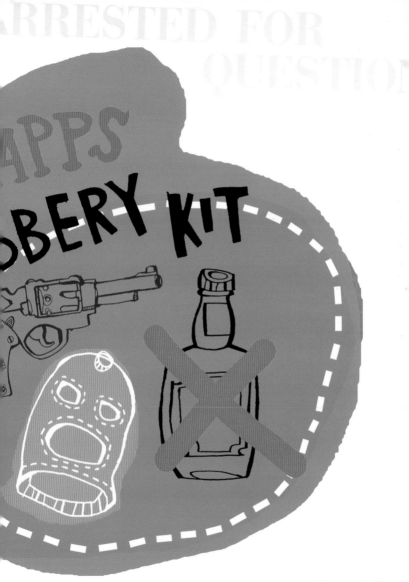

FUNNY, I THOUGHT PIT BULLS WERE BIGGER THAN THIS

IRVINE | Calif   REUTERS

They thought they had stolen vicious pit bulls but instead they wound up with purse-sized Chihuahua dogs.

Two men were arrested for stealing the puppies from an animal shelter in this southern California city a couple of days earlier.

The men were caught after bringing the dogs, which had ID microchips implanted under their skin, to an animal clinic in a PetSmart pet supply store for an examination and vaccinations.

The store's director said she recognized the puppies and the suspects from their descriptions on a flier she received from the animal shelter.

The store manager said she sensed that the pups were victims of a severe case of mistaken identity. "They asked me, 'What is this?'" she said. "I told them it looked like a Chihuahua mix. They said, 'No way, it's a pit bull.' They didn't believe me. They wanted to ask the veterinarian.

"They were pretty perturbed that the puppies they stole were not pit bulls," the manager said. "They thought they were stealing pit bulls. These guys are idiots," the pet store manager said.

it looked like a Chihuahua mix.

Kids, Don't Try This At Home

WICHITA | Kan   REUTERS

A Kansas man who got a coat hanger stuck in his throat while trying to dislodge a balloon of cocaine he had swallowed faced possible criminal charges after doctors trying to remove the hanger discovered the drugs, police said.

According to police, the man decided to stick the hooked end of a coat hanger into his throat in an effort to retrieve a small balloon he said he accidentally swallowed while at a party.

"He just bent it and forced it down his throat," said a police spokeswoman.

The hooked end of the hanger became lodged in the man's throat and he was rushed to a Wichita-area hospital where doctors initially were baffled by the bizarre circumstances, police said.

But in operating on the man to remove the hanger, police said surgeons found the drug-filled balloon.

The man was expected to remain hospitalized for more than a week but was expected to recover. Police said they were recommending to prosecutors that the 33-year-old man be charged with felony possession of cocaine.

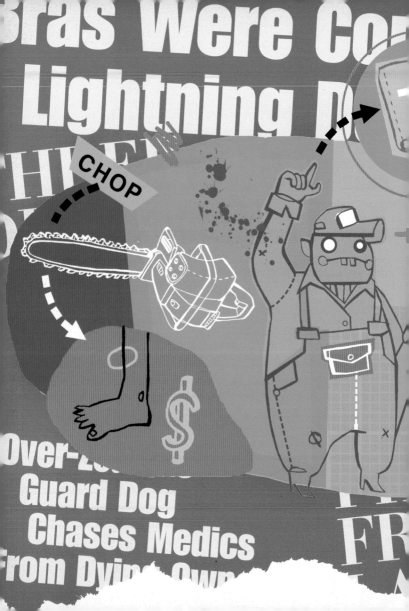

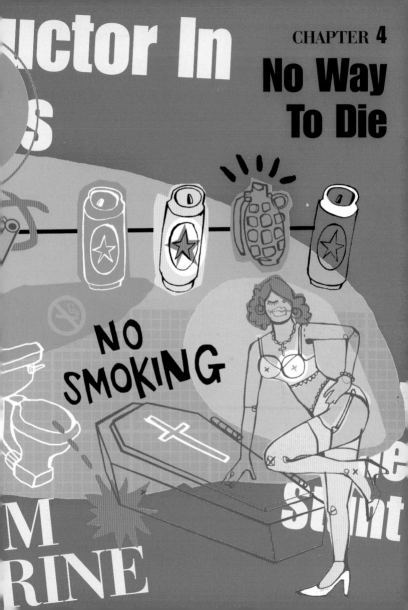

INSURANCE SCAM TURNS INTO CHAINSAW HORROR

ROME   REUTERS

An Italian man is accused of killing his cousin with a chainsaw in a billion lire ($460,000) insurance scam that went horribly wrong.

Justice sources said the body of a 23-year-old man was discovered in a pool of blood in his hometown in the far north of Italy.

They said his 29-year-old cousin insisted that the death was a genuine accident.

The sources said the accused wanted to cash in on a generous insurance policy and had persuaded his cousin to cut open his leg with a chainsaw. To make it look like a crime, the cousin then fled the scene and threw the chainsaw into a nearby river.

The victim, a part-time bouncer who wanted to become a private detective, was a first aid expert and the pair believed he would be able to stem the bleeding before calling for help.

But the cut was too deep and when he phoned for an ambulance his voice was so distorted by pain operators could not understand where he was.

The cousin was under arrest and faces a murder charge.

man was
discovered
in a pool of blood

Guard Dog Chases Medics From Dying Owner

MOSCOW   REUTERS

A Russian man paid the price for training his guard dog too well when the snarling animal held off paramedics long enough for him to die of heart failure.

The ferocious Staffordshire bull terrier kept doctors at bay as they tried to approach the middle-aged patient.

"Doctors and the man's wife tried to approach the man for a long time, but the dog was furious and would not allow it," a regional police chief said by telephone from the city of Chelyabinsk near the Ural mountains.

"The doctors had to call the police, and our officers shot the dog, but by the time the doctors could get in, the patient was dead."

Bras Act As Conductor

LONDON   REUTERS

Two women were killed by a bolt of lightning in London's Hyde Park when their underwire bras acted as conductors, a coroner said.

"I think this was a tragic case, a pure act of God," the coroner told an inquest into the deaths. He recorded a verdict of death by misadventure.

"This is only the second time in my experience of 50,000 deaths where lightning has struck the metal in a bra causing death, but I do not wish to over-emphasize any significance," the coroner said. The two women had been sheltering under a tree in the park during a thunderstorm.

A pathologist said both women were wearing underwire bras and had been left with burn marks on their chests from the electrical current.

THREE DIE RETRIEVING PHONE FROM LATRINE

NAIROBI   REUTERS

Three Kenyans died trying to retrieve a mobile phone that slipped down an open-pit latrine while its owner answered a call of nature, a newspaper reported.

Anxious to recover her phone, the owner in the coastal town of Mombasa offered 1,000 shillings ($13.09) to anyone who would recover it, the *Daily Nation* said.

Well over half the Kenyan population of 30 million people lives on less than $1 a day.

The first to try—a 30-year-old radio technician—failed to resurface after disappearing down a ladder into the latrine.

His friend went after him but slipped and fell. The third casualty, trying to rescue the others, was hauled out of the pit by neighbors after he inhaled the fumes and lost consciousness.

The man was rushed to hospital but died on the way.

"The fumes inside must be extremely poisonous considering the short time it was taking to disable the retrievers," acting Mombasa police chief Peter Njenga was reported as saying.

The *Daily Nation* said police prevented a fourth man from climbing into the latrine and the search for the phone was eventually abandoned.

HOIST WITH HIS OWN PETARD?

BRUSSELS   REUTERS

A Belgian man died of a gunshot wound after setting booby traps throughout his house using hunting rifles and explosives, police and local news reports said.

The 80-year-old former chemical engineer had apparently set the traps to prevent his children from entering the house after a family dispute, the local Belga news agency said.

Police, who had worked from before dawn searching and dismantling the traps, had yet to determine whether the man died from self-inflicted wounds or one of his own traps, it said.

The traps throughout the house were set to go off with the opening of a door or some other makeshift trigger, the officer said.

Talking To The Dead

LONDON   REUTERS

Two British mental health workers visited a patient, chatted with her and then left without realizing she was dead, newspapers said.

An inquest heard that the workers from the mental health charity Mind let themselves into the home of a paranoid schizophrenic and found her sitting in the kitchen with the curtains drawn and her back to them.

They left when she failed to respond, the *Daily Mail* reported. "She didn't seem to want us there," a health worker was quoted as saying.

The next day, two other health workers on a visit discovered she was dead.

Death, Where Is Thy Sting?

ROME   REUTERS

Death is hardly something to look forward to, but one Italian funeral home is trying to make the afterlife a tad more tempting by using bikini-clad women to sell its coffins.

On its Web site, the Rome-based funeral home and coffin factory features its hand-crafted caskets alongside models sipping champagne or reclining seductively on the lids.

"We wanted to make the whole idea of picking your coffin less serious, maybe even make people laugh a bit," one of the partners said.

Near-naked women are used to sell everything in Italy from computers to chocolate bars, but this firm has taken the advertising ploy to new limits.

The page featuring the firm's "Madonna" coffin shows a pouting woman in zebra shorts and high-heel boots kneeling next to the casket, while in "Empire Style," a blonde donning a black G-string leans on a coffin and turns her backside to the camera.

black
g-string

"MADONNA" CC

SOMEBODY YOU DON'T WANT TO DRINK WITH

KIEV REUTERS

A Ukrainian woman in Donetsk was blown to pieces when she pulled the pin out of a hand grenade which she had mistaken for a can of beer, the Ukrinform news agency said.

Local police chief Stanislav Gavrilenko told the agency that 17 people were also injured when the woman accidentally detonated the hand grenade near the city's railway station.

Ukrainian police were carrying out a major search for illegal weapons and Gavrilenko said the grenade had probably been thrown away by a suspect on the run.

Fiery Summer Snowmobile Stunt

VANCOUVER | British Columbia REUTERS

A Canadian man who tried to drive his snowmobile through a ball of flames during a drunken summer party has died of his injuries, police said.

The man was severely burned in the tragic incident in Squamish, British Columbia.

Witnesses told police the 23-year-old rode the snowmobile in a "wheelie" down a paved public street and tried to drive it through a gasoline fire at the end of the run.

Local media reported his stunt was also being recorded for use in a video of extreme sports events.

Freak Pea Drop Kills Man

STOCKHOLM   REUTERS

A Swedish man died when he was buried alive under a 13-ton pile of peas in a storage silo, local media reported.

The man, who was around 30 years old, was working on an electrical installation on a farm near the town of Mjolby in southeastern Sweden when the peas were dumped on him.

Rescue workers pulled the man out from the silo but were unable to revive him according to the local radio station.

MAN DIES VISITING HIS FUTURE GRAVE

LASCARI | Sicily   REUTERS

An Italian man sent himself, literally, to an early grave.

The 63-year-old man was so keen that his future mausoleum would be a perfect fit that he liked to visit it to ensure the builders were making it just right.

But his latest visit proved to be his last.

According to local media reports, the man was making his regular trip to the construction site in the small cemetery in his hometown.

He climbed a ladder to get a better view of the top of the mausoleum when he slipped, hit his head on a marble step, and fell into his own tomb.

HAS THIS EVER HAPPENED TO YOU?

RIO DE JANEIRO | Brazil   REUTERS

Bones, coffins and crosses crashed through the kitchen wall of a Brazilian home over the weekend after a torrential rain washed out part of a neighboring cemetery, officials said.

"It happened during the rain Saturday night. Part of the cemetery wall fell and earth mixed with body parts, coffins and pieces of tombstones invaded the house that is located down the hill," said an official at the cemetery on the outskirts of Rio de Janeiro who did not want to be named.

Cemetery officials said the residents had to tolerate the remnants of the dead in their kitchen for the rest of the weekend. A funeral home in the area was expected to clean up the "haunted" house Monday.

The residents could not be reached for comment. Brazil's *Extra* tabloid newspaper showed a picture of a woman living in the house holding up a hip bone and a piece of a skull, with a pile of earth and a huge opening in a wall in the background.

Bones, coffins and crosses

Wife Killed Over "Disgusting Coffee"

ROME   REUTERS

An Italian man said he had killed his 72-year-old wife after she made him a bad cup of coffee, Italian news agency ANSA reported.

"The coffee was disgusting. I drank a little then I picked up the cup and smashed it on the floor," the 84-year-old told prosecutors in Bari, on Italy's southern heel, the agency said.

"My wife screamed and I slapped her. Then I grabbed the hammer and hit her," the man said.

A neighbor discovered the wife's body and alerted the police. The man was arrested on suspicion of murder.

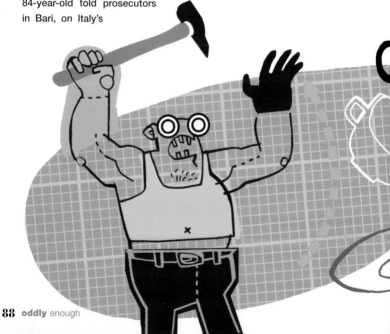

NOW, ONE OF THEM KNOWS THE ANSWER...

GODLEY | Texas   REUTERS

An argument over who was going to heaven and who was going to hell ended with one Texas man shooting another to death with a shotgun, police said.

The two had spent Saturday with two other men bar-hopping in Fort Worth, about 40 miles northeast of Godley.

The Johnson County sheriff said a witness who was the designated driver for the group told police the four men were sitting at a table outside a trailer park after their night on the town and entered into an argument about religion. The talk became heated when the subject turned to who would go to heaven and who would go to hell.

One of the men said he would settle the argument and went into a house and returned with a shotgun, which he loaded and placed in his mouth, the sheriff said the witness reported.

"The victim then took the gun out of the man's mouth, saying, 'If you have to shoot somebody, shoot me,'" the sheriff said, citing the witness report.

The shotgun went off, hitting the victim in the chest and killing him.

KILLERS FED DISMEMBERED VICTIM TO LIONS

JOHANNESBURG   REUTERS

Two South Africans who killed the daughter of a creditor, dismembered her body and then fed it to lions were handed life sentences by a Johannesburg court, a newspaper reported.

The two had kidnapped the woman, to whose mother one of them owed money, and asked for 200,000 rand ($21,100) for her return, the paper said.

They received 80,000 rand of that, but killed the 23-year-old woman anyway, disposing of her body in a lion park to the north of Johannesburg.

The *Daily Star* reported that a High Court judge had given the two killers life sentences, quoting him as saying their acts reached a level of cruelty not seen before in the country's courts.

"In order to conceal their dastardly act, one of two of the accused dismembered the victim, boiled the body and disseminated the body, presumably for the consumption of lions," the paper quoted the judge as saying. It said a few of the victim's vertebrae and ribs were recovered from the park.

Two Charged After Human Catapult Death

LONDON   REUTERS

British police charged two men with manslaughter following the death of an Oxford University student who was flung from a giant catapult.

The 19-year-old student died when the stunt near the West Country town of Bridgewater went wrong.

"He had been thrown by a replica medieval catapult and failed to reach the landing net," said a police spokeswoman.

The student was on an outing with the Oxford Stunt Factory, an unofficial club at Oxford University where he was studying biochemistry. He had been the sixth person that day to be launched from the "trebuchet" catapult.

Organizers said at the time he had been properly weighed and that the machine had been correctly calibrated before he was fired in a 30-yard arc. They did not know what had gone wrong.

Exploding Toilet Kills Man

BONN   REUTERS

A German camper died from injuries received when a campsite toilet exploded as he tried to light a cigarette. The explosion managed to blast him through a closed window, police said.

Police in the town of Montabaur south of Bonn said the explosion appeared to have been caused by leaking gas from the septic tank or a defective natural gas pipe.

The 32-year-old man was taken to a hospital suffering from burns and died.

Grenade Blast Kills Four At Wedding Party

PHNOM PENH REUTERS

A hand-grenade carried by a guest at a Cambodian wedding party fell off his belt as he was dancing and exploded, killing four people and injuring 41, officials said.

The governor of Prey Veng province in eastern Cambodia said the teenager appeared to be showing off to impress his girlfriend when the grenade exploded.

"The bride and groom are very lucky because they were tired and went to their bedroom before the tragedy happened," he said.

The man carrying the grenade was among those killed.

NAP ON A HOT TIN ROOF

BERLIN REUTERS

High temperatures sweeping Germany claimed an unlikely victim when a man sleeping on a roof to escape the heat rolled off, suffering fatal injuries, Berlin police said.

A tenant of the building found the 28-year-old still alive after his 70-foot fall, but he later died in hospital. The man had bedded down with two friends as temperatures neared 86 degrees in the German capital.

The friends only learned of the man's fate after being awakened and informed by police.

"The man must have ended up on the steep part of the roof and fallen off," Berlin police said in a statement.

His sleeping bag remained hanging off the gutter at the edge of the tiled roof.

Man Dies After Decapitation Attempt

BRATISLAVA   REUTERS

A Slovak man died after trying to decapitate himself with a homemade guillotine because he had fallen behind in paying his taxes, police said.

The 56-year-old man drove his car in front of the tax office in the western Slovak town of Malacky late last month, pulled out a device resembling a guillotine, stuck his head in it and tried to decapitate himself, the police said.

"It did not cut his head off completely ... but he wounded himself so badly that he died afterwards," the Malacky police chief told Reuters.

The man left a message, saying he could no longer pay his taxes, which totaled around 25,000 crowns ($542).

HOMEMADE GUILLOTINE

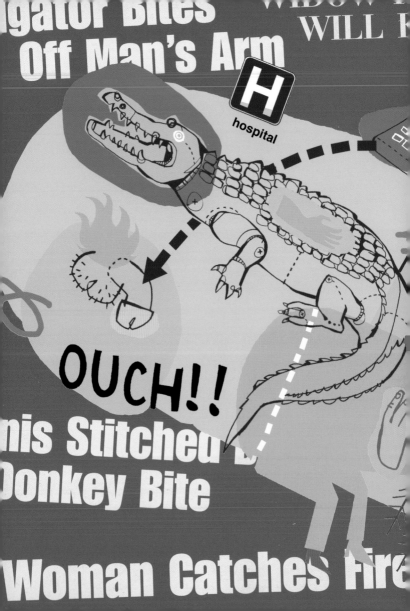

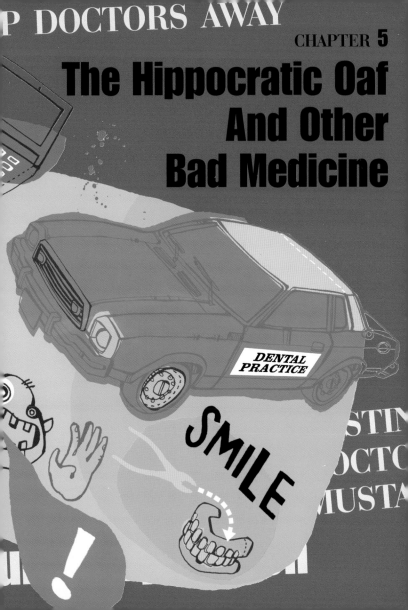

Woman Catches Fire During Operation

WELLINGTON   REUTERS

A woman caught fire while undergoing a Caesarean operation at a New Zealand hospital, media reported.

The woman was on the operating table at Auckland's Waitakere Hospital with the baby still in her womb when the fire broke out, the *New Zealand Herald* reported.

Medical staff smothered the flames but the mother—who had been given an epidural partial anesthetic—suffered burns to the lower part of her body, the newspaper said.

Her baby boy was delivered unharmed.

Investigations into the cause of the freak accident centered on an alcohol-based swabbing solution used to sterilize the woman's abdomen for the surgery.

Equipment used to cut through skin and cauterize bleeding may have ignited the swabbing solution, investigators told the *Herald*.

A spokeswoman for the public hospital said the hospital had switched to a non-alcohol swabbing solution while the accident was being investigated.

BUSTING DOCTOR MUSTANG...

MIAMI REUTERS

Florida police have arrested a man who allegedly ran a mobile dentistry practice from the back of his dilapidated 1980 Ford Mustang.

The suspect used homemade drills he failed to sterilize and set up a dental lab in his efficiency apartment, which was strewn with rusty car parts, a police spokesman in Hialeah, Florida, said.

The man was arrested after an undercover agent sought him out to remove an ailing molar. Police swept in before the agent lost any teeth, said a police spokesman.

They set up the sting after getting calls from people reporting "very strange and weird activity ... Someone performing dental and medical work in his vehicle," the spokesman said.

The "dentist" practiced in Hialeah, a blue-collar city west of Miami, and mainly treated poor, Spanish-speaking patients who thought his $30 to $60 fees were a bargain, police said.

He was charged with practicing dentistry without a license, illegal possession of regulated drugs and running an unregistered dental laboratory.

Police said the suspect had no dental or medical training.

suspect used
homemade drills

Doctor Performs Brain Surgery With Store Drill

LIMA   REUTERS

Lacking the proper instruments, a Peruvian doctor at a state hospital in the Andean highlands used a drill and pliers to perform brain surgery on a man who had been injured in a fight, the doctor said.

"We have no (neurosurgical) instruments at the hospital. He was dying, so I had no choice but to run to a hardware store to buy a drill and use the pliers that I fix my car with, of course after sterilizing them," the doctor told Reuters in a telephone interview.

The patient had arrived at the hospital in Andahuaylas, 240 miles southeast of Lima, after being hit in the head with a metal object in a street fight, the doctor said.

"I drilled holes in his skull in a circle, leaving spaces of 5 millimeters, took out the bone with the pliers and removed the clots that were putting pressure on his brain," he said.

The doctor, who earns $430 a month, said he had used tools from a hardware store on five previous occasions but for less serious operations.

The patient was making a good recovery in a hospital.

STRESS RELIEF STRESSES NEIGHBORS

AACHEN REUTERS

A man who relieved his stress by repeatedly entering a forest to scream has been ordered to find a different way to relax because he was scaring neighbors, German police said.

Residents in the western town of Aachen called police to investigate a series of loud yells coming from a local forest.

"We found a 25-year-old man who said walking into the forest at night alone and screaming as loudly as he could was his way of dealing with the stress of everyday life," said a police spokesman.

The man's screams had prompted neighbors to call police out on three previous occasions.

He now faces a fine of 75 euros (dollars). "That stressed him out again but officers told him not to go in the forest this time," the spokesman said.

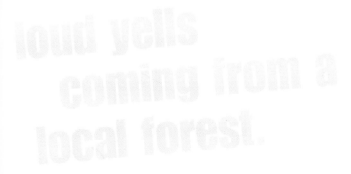

loud yells coming from a local forest.

Alligator Bites Off Man's Arm

MIAMI   REUTERS

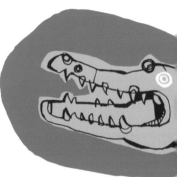

An 11-foot bull alligator tore off a man's arm and swallowed it at a north Florida botanical garden, wildlife officials said.

Trappers killed the alligator and recovered the severed arm from its stomach but doctors said it was too badly mangled to try reattaching it.

The injured man was listed in fair condition at Shands Hospital at the University of Florida where he was "in good spirits," a spokeswoman said.

The victim was weeding a lily pond, standing in about four feet of water, when he apparently stepped straight on the 392-pound male alligator, a captain from the Florida Fish and Wildlife Conservation Commission said.

The alligator "lunged up and grabbed hold of his right arm and severed it just below the elbow," he added.

The victim climbed out of the pond and shouted for a co-worker, who took off his shirt and fashioned it into a tourniquet to help staunch the bleeding until paramedics arrived.

Trappers harpooned the alligator and hoisted it to the bank, where a sheriff's deputy shot it in the head with a 12-gauge shotgun and killed it, said the captain.

"I physically slit the alligator open, reached in, and I could feel the victim's arm in the stomach," he told Reuters by phone. "I was able to sever the stomach and pull the victim's arm out."

The arm was recovered about 90 minutes after the attack, he said. Paramedics took it to the hospital but it was too badly damaged to be reattached.

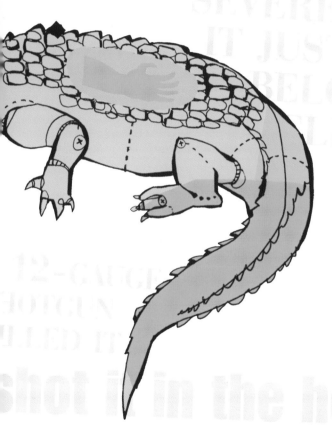

FAKE SURGEON ACCUSED OF MANGLING PATIENTS

MIAMI REUTERS

Miami Beach police said they were looking for a fake doctor who drugged people with an animal anesthetic and performed botched cosmetic surgeries that left one man with female breast implants and a woman with badly misshapen breasts.

Police said the suspect had no medical training.

Two other people have been arrested in connection with the bizarre case—one who delivered the anesthetic and another who assisted in the operations.

All three face charges of practicing medicine without a license, aggravated battery and improper use of a controlled substance, the anesthetic.

Authorities began investigating after a patient, described as a former model in her 20s, showed them a videotape she had made of the fake doctor allegedly operating on a male body builder who wanted pectoral implants.

"He ended up with female breast implants," police Capt. Charles Press said.

According to Press, the tape showed the "doctor" jamming the implants into the patient's chest with "a spatula-type thing that you'd see in a kitchen" and sewing up the incision with crude X-shaped stitches.

The patient awoke three times during the procedure and was told to go back to sleep, he said.

"This was a horror movie," Press said. "They did things to this guy that would just boggle the mind."

Scientist Burns Penis With Laptop

LONDON   REUTERS

Laptops have always been a hot item but a 50-year-old scientist didn't realize to what extent until he burned his penis.

The previously healthy father of two reported feeling a burning sensation after he had been writing a report at home for about an hour with the laptop computer resting on his lap.

He noticed a redness and irritation the following day but it wasn't until he was examined by a doctor that he realized how much damage had been done.

"The ventral part of his scrotal skin had turned red, and there was a blister with a diameter of about two centimeters (0.8 inches)," said a letter published in *The Lancet* medical journal.

Two days later, the blisters broke and the wounds became infected and then crusted but after about a week the unidentified scientist was "healing quite rapidly."

HIS SCROTAL SKIN HAD TURNED RED

BROKEN LEG MAKES MAN MILLIONAIRE

MELBOURNE   REUTERS

An Australian man nursing a broken leg has become a millionaire by picking lottery-winning numbers from his hospital identification bracelet.

The Melbourne man split a A$3.0 million ($1.5 million) prize pool with two other winners from New South Wales and Queensland states.

The unidentified man in his 50s said he wrote the numbers on his lottery ticket after looking at the registration number written on his hospital bracelet.

A source at the hospital confirmed the agency's report but declined to give further details.

Penis Stitched Back After Donkey Bite

RABAT   REUTERS

Surgeons have managed to stitch back a Moroccan boy's penis after it was bitten off by a donkey, the official MAP news agency reported.

The chief urologist at Ibnou Toufail Hospital in the southern city of Marrakesh was quoted as saying that the successful operation on the seven-year-old boy took a total of 45 minutes.

MAP did not say how the donkey managed to bite off the boy's penis.

Man Sues Doctor Who Left Surgery To Cash Check

BOSTON   REUTERS

A Massachusetts man filed a malpractice lawsuit against the doctor who left him on the operating table midway through spinal surgery to cash a check at a nearby bank.

The patient said he suffers severe pain in his right leg after the orthopedic surgeon left him for 35 minutes with an open incision in his back during a spinal fusion procedure at a Boston-area hospital. His lawyer filed the lawsuit in Suffolk County Superior Court in Boston.

The surgeon, whose license to practice medicine was suspended by the state medical board, has acknowledged that he temporarily abandoned the patient in the operating room during the operation at Mount Auburn Hospital in Cambridge, Massachusetts.

The doctor admitted to a medical board investigator that he had "exercised remarkably horrible judgment" during the surgery, according to a board report.

The surgeon explained to the investigator he had been waiting for his paycheck because he had to pay some overdue bills and had been hoping to finish the surgery before his bank closed for the day.

The procedure took longer than he expected, however, and he decided to make a break for the bank midway through surgery.

Hope You Like The Necklace, Honey...Guess Where It Came From

BOCA RATON | Fla.   REUTERS

A 16-inch diamond necklace apparently swallowed by a jewel thief was put up for auction on the Internet by its owner, who hopes to cash in on the gems' unusual journey.

Police said they recovered the necklace, studded with 83 diamonds, from a man who was charged with grand theft after X-rays showed the missing necklace and two loose diamonds in his digestive system.

The incident was widely reported by the news media and the necklace became the butt of jokes on the talk shows, prompting a flood of phone calls to the shop in Boca Raton.

"We have been getting so much attention over the matter, we decided to auction the item on eBay," the storeowner said.

He set the minimum bid at $75,000 for the necklace, which contains nearly 30 carats of diamonds. He said he expected it to sell for well over $100,000 in the 10-day auction.

The necklace has been sterilized, boiled and cleaned with alcohol and jewelry cleaner.

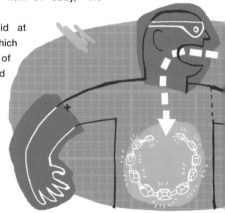

WIDOW HOPES TATTOO WILL KEEP DOCTORS AWAY

LONDON   REUTERS

An 85-year-old widow is so determined not to be resuscitated against her will by doctors that she has tattooed the words "Do Not Resuscitate" across her chest.

The woman, a former nurse, said she paid $40 for a tattoo with the instruction and a heart with a "no-go" sign to ensure medical staff knew she did not want to be revived.

"Years ago when I was nursing I could see they resuscitated so many people they shouldn't have," she told reporters at the *Nursing Standard* magazine.

"I don't want to die twice. By resuscitating me, they would be bringing me back from the dead only for me to have to go through it again," she said.

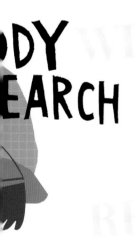

staff forgot to hook up the machine

BLUNDER LEAVES WOMAN AWAKE DURING SURGERY

VIENNA   REUTERS

A woman lay awake during surgery for 45 minutes, unable to move or call for help, after staff forgot to hook up the machine pumping out anesthetic, the Austrian daily *Kurier* reported.

The woman was temporarily paralyzed because she had been given a muscle relaxant, and her ordeal ended only after a replacement doctor who came into the operating room saw tears in her eyes and noticed the machine was not connected properly.

The woman, who was undergoing abdominal surgery, is suing for 70,000 euros ($79,970) in damages, the hospital in the Austrian province of Carinthia confirmed.

Two Charged With Glue Dentistry

MIAMI · REUTERS

Two flea market jewelers were arrested on charges of practicing dentistry without a license after an undercover investigation found they were gluing gold inlays to people's teeth from the back of their 10-year-old Honda.

Word-of-mouth marketing drew several customers a day who flipped through a photo album of styles before bargaining over the cost of the cosmetic procedure that could range from $150 to $1,000, investigators said.

"They could give you a whole rack of gold, or just cover a few teeth. They even had gold vampire fangs, if that's what you wanted," said a spokesman for the Broward Sheriff's Department.

Men Opt For Penis Extensions, Clinic Says

LONDON REUTERS

Penis extensions are the top cosmetic surgery treatment for British men while women choose liposuction or breast enlargement, medics said.

The Harley Medical Group, which runs 10 private clinics in Britain, released figures for 2002 which showed more than a third of operations on men were for penis extensions, followed by nose surgery and liposuction.

Men made up 35 percent of the group's patients last year and their average age was 22–37 years old.

Alien Halloween No Child's Play For Paramedics

LONDON　　REUTERS

A group of British paramedics had the fright of their lives this Halloween, when they mistook a child's toy found on a London subway station platform for a human fetus and rushed it to hospital.

Officials closed down Buckhurst Hill station in Essex, northwest of London, on Halloween night, fearing a woman had had a miscarriage, a London Underground spokeswoman said.

They had found an alien egg toy, which unbeknown to them was the latest toy craze to hit the London area. It contained what looked like a tiny unborn child curled in a fetal position and suspended in a gooey placenta-like substance.

"Paramedics thought the toy alien was a human fetus, and the mistake was only discovered when it was examined in hospital," explained the Underground spokeswoman.

CATS GET GO-AHEAD FOR KIDNEY TRANSPLANT

LONDON REUTERS

The British, long ridiculed for pampering their pets, can now indulge their cats with a costly kidney transplant.

The Royal College of Veterinary Surgeons said it has given the go-ahead for the operation after its success in the United States prompted British cat lovers to demand the right to transplants.

"We are not encouraging transplantation or opposing it but we want to make sure that there are guidelines in place for the profession to be able to follow," an external relations officer at the college told Reuters.

The operation will come at a price.

In the United States, cat kidney transplants have cost between $7,000 and $10,000, and vets estimate the cost in Britain at between 8,000 and 10,000 pounds ($12,600 and $15,800).

Even so, the procedure will extend a cat's life by an average of only two years and in most cases the cat will remain on medication for the rest of its life. The rise of kidney transplants for pets has caused uproar among animal welfare groups who fear the lives of strays will be sacrificed to keep much-loved pets alive.

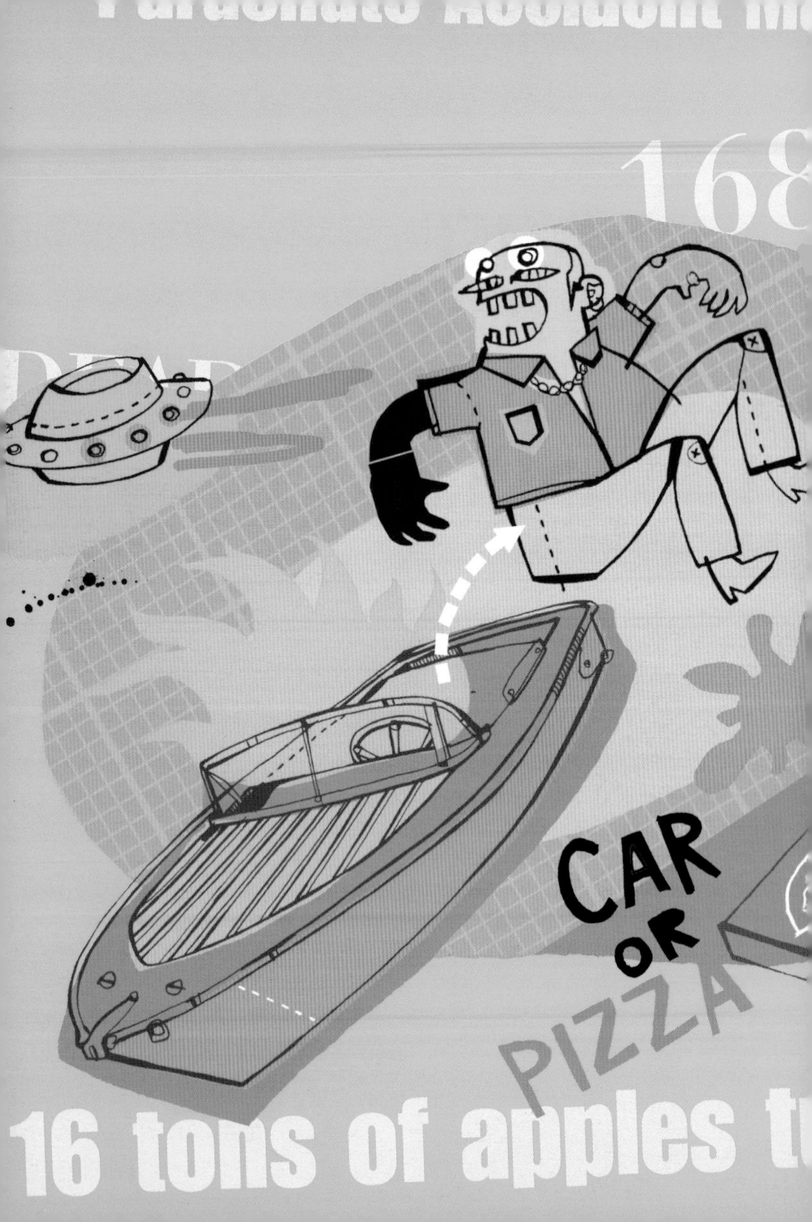
168
CAR
OR
PIZZA
16 tons of apples

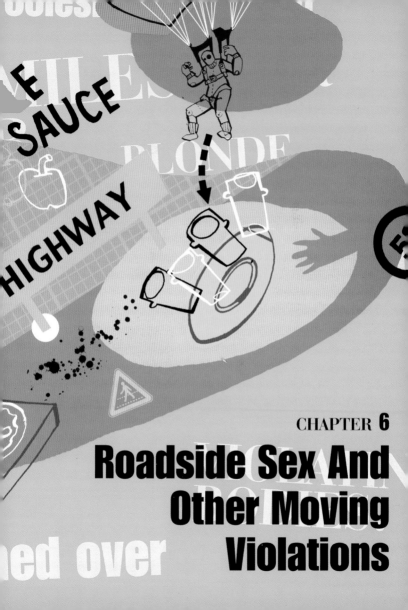

CHAPTER **6**

Roadside Sex And Other Moving Violations

Parachute Accident Mars Coleslaw Wrestling

SAMSALA | Fla.   REUTERS

A parachutist landed on a beer vendor at a coleslaw wrestling match during central Florida's raucous "Bike Week" celebration, seriously injuring the vendor, sheriff's deputies said.

The accident occurred at Sopotnick's Cabbage Patch bar in Samsala, which sponsors an annual coleslaw wrestling match as part of the motorcycle festival that draws as many as 500,000 riders from around the nation to the Daytona Beach area.

Just before the women wrestlers squared off in a pit full of cabbage and oil, a sky diver hired to parachute into the makeshift arena was blown off course by high winds.

"The parachutist missed his mark and landed on top of the victim," a Volusia County Sheriff's spokesman said. The victim was walking with a tray full of beer near the beverage concession, where she and other members of a local charity were working.

"We yelled, 'Move, dummy!' but she never looked up because it happened so quick," a biker told the *Orlando Sentinel*.

The victim suffered head and facial injuries and was taken by helicopter to Halifax Medical Center, where she was reported to be in serious but stable condition.

The parachutist, who said he never saw the woman, said the impact "knocked the wind out of me" but he was uninjured.

"Knocked The Wind Out Of Me"

BIG CRASH ON "APPLE SAUCE" HIGHWAY

PADERBORN | Germany   REUTERS

A major German motorway was closed unexpectedly for several hours after a truck carrying 16 tons of apples turned over, transforming the Autobahn 33 into a hazardous apple sauce skidpan.

Police said three cars drove into the slush formed by thousands of smashed apples strewn over a 500-yard section of the motorway near the western town of Paderborn, and crashed into two trucks. One woman was slightly injured.

"It was a miracle there wasn't a major pileup," a police spokesman said, adding that the apple sauce was about four inches thick and looked like fresh snow. Firefighters used snowplows and shovels to clear the motorway.

So, Like, I Didn't Pass The Test?

AMSTERDAM   REUTERS

A man was forced to abandon his driving test when his car became stuck at a railway crossing and was ripped apart by two trains.

The 22-year-old and his driving examiner made a hurried escape from the car when its engine cut out as it straddled the railway tracks near The Hague, police said.

The car was first dragged 150 yards along the rails by one train, then pulled the other way by a train heading in the opposite direction.

No one was injured, but train services between The Hague and Rotterdam were severely delayed.

ripped apart by
two trains

WRONG COLOR CAR SAVES CRIME VICTIM

JOHANNESBURG   REUTERS

Being hijacked to one of South Africa's urban slums can be a death sentence for motorists, but having the wrong color car saved a Johannesburg woman and her children.

The would-be recipient of her Swedish saloon car complained that it was the wrong color, prompting the hijackers to give the woman her keys back and tell her to leave—after giving her directions.

Police said the woman, whom they declined to name, was surprised at her garden gate shortly after dark by three armed men, who forced her into the backseat of the white car with her son and daughter, aged 14 and nine.

The hijackers drove her to Alexandra, an inner-city slum where police are as rare as street lights. She then had to wait in the car while one of the hijackers talked to their client.

"The client apparently said the car was the wrong color. But the amazing thing was that the hijackers then gave the woman her keys back and told her to leave," a police spokeswoman told Reuters.

They only asked for her mobile phone and some jewelry, which she gave them, the spokeswoman said. Then they gave her detailed directions after she said she did not know how to get out of Alexandra.

They only asked f her mobile phone

High-Speed Nap Gets Engineer In Trouble

TOKYO   REUTERS

A Japanese bullet-train driver has brought new meaning to the phrase "a quick nap."

The 33-year-old, whose name has not been released, was being questioned by police after falling asleep for about eight minutes at the controls of one of the country's high-speed bullet trains.

West Japan Railways said the train may have been traveling at up to 168 miles per hour while the driver was slumbering.

No one was hurt because an automatic control system kicked in, eventually bringing the train to a halt.

The incident came to light after the dozing driver was awakened by a conductor.

"We are very shocked," said Kosuke Sugiyama of the company's public relations office. "Our business is all about passengers trusting us enough to travel on our trains."

Japan's bullet trains have a reputation for punctuality timed to the second and drivers are highly trained.

Guy Admits Driving On "20 Beers At Most"

BERLIN   REUTERS

An inebriated German driver's honesty cost him his license after he told police he had drunk "20 beers at most," authorities said.

During a routine traffic check in the western city of Essen, police asked if the 25-year-old man driving his car had drunk anything in the past few hours. He didn't hesitate to answer:

"Twenty beers at most if you want me to be perfectly honest, officer. But that's it, really."

Police carried out a breath test, confirming the man's claims, and confiscated his license. "I've no idea why he told them," said a spokesman for Essen police. "Maybe because he was drunk."

LIKE FATHER, LIKE SON AS POLICE NAB DRIVERS

BERLIN   REUTERS

A German father and son both lost their driving licenses within hours of each other for being drunk at the wheel of a car.

First of all the son was caught and then the inebriated father tried to help out by going to pick him up, police said.

"First the son came off the road under the influence, so police took his license. Then the father set off for the scene of the accident, got stopped and was also found to be over the limit, so he had his taken too," said a police spokesman in the southern town of Hildesheim.

STOWAWAYS TAKE ROUND TRIP

BOGOTA | Colombia   REUTERS

Yelling "Hey, Colombian people!" five Colombian stowaways emerged jubilantly from a ship they thought had docked in Miami only to discover they were still in their homeland after five days at sea, police said.

The Dutch-flagged cargo ship carrying the unfortunate five, which sailed from Buenaventura on Sunday, had mechanical problems, which meant that its five-day journey only took it as far as another Colombian port, Cartagena.

The stowaways' rudimentary English yells of joy were interrupted when they were arrested by Colombian police.

"They wanted the American dream, but they only made it to Cartagena," said the director of the local branch of the DAS detective force, adding that two of the men had previous records as stowaways.

Looking sheepish and giggling, the five were paraded in front of local reporters before being freed and put on a bus back to Buenaventura.

"Hey, Colombian people!"

Fuel Crunch Leads To Rent-A-Corpse Scam

HARARE   REUTERS

Two Zimbabwean mortuary workers have been arrested on charges they rented out corpses to motorists to enable them to take advantage of special fuel preferences given to hearses.

Zimbabwe's state-owned *Herald* newspaper reported that a mortician and an assistant at a public hospital were arrested and would soon appear in court on charges of violating dead bodies.

The two were accused of running a racket under which they sold fake burial orders to motorists who then took the corpses and transported them to service stations.

That allowed them to jump long lines to fill their tanks.

After buying the fuel they returned the bodies in their coffins to the mortuary, the newspaper said.

Smugglers Burn Boat—Not Cocaine

BOGOTA | Colombia   REUTERS

Their plan was to burn cocaine valued at $75 million before the Colombian navy reached their speedboat—far, far off the country's Pacific coast.

Instead, the quick-thinking drug traffickers had to jump ship when their boat caught fire. To their surprise, the bagged cocaine also spilled into the ocean—and some even was found bobbing alongside the crew when authorities arrived.

"When they saw themselves surrounded, the crew of the boat set a fire to erase the evidence. But the boat didn't burn completely and some packets of the drug wound up floating," the navy said in a statement.

The navy added that it "rescued" the five crew members, who were subsequently arrested and brought to shore.

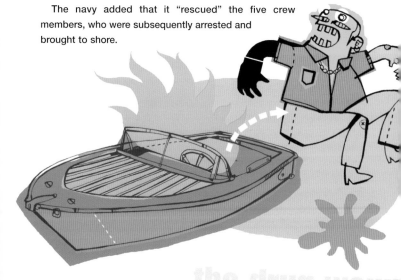

PARACHUTES FOR OFFICE WORKERS

JERUSALEM REUTERS

An Israeli company has designed a parachute for workers in high-rise buildings in the aftermath of the suicide-hijacking attacks that toppled the World Trade Center.

"Within three weeks of the attack, the Executivechute was designed, tested and ready to go," Anatoly Cohen, managing director of Apco Aviation, said. The backpack-type parachute, which is being marketed in the United States and Japan, has a $795 price tag and weighs four pounds.

Its rip cord can be attached to heavy furniture or a special hook so that the parachute opens automatically after its wearer jumps out a window.

The military-style round canopy, as opposed to an aerobatic rectangular design, makes for a reliable but hard landing from a minimum height of 10 stories.

"It's unlikely the user will know how to do the standard 'paratroop roll' upon hitting the ground," Cohen told Reuters. "But we figure a twisted ankle is a small price to pay for life."

Boy Run Over By Truck He Stole

OVERLAND PARK | Kan.　　**REUTERS**

A 17-year-old was run over by the pickup truck he had stolen, police said.

The teenager, whose name was not released because he was a juvenile, caught the attention of police as the pickup wove through the streets of Overland Park, a south Kansas City-area suburb.

Police were able to coax the driver into stopping the vehicle, but he jumped from the truck and tried to make a run for it.

"The vehicle began to roll just as the driver ducked in front of it," said a policeman. "He stumbled and fell and the truck ran over him."

The suspect was hospitalized with minor injuries.

HER ARM CAUGHT, WOMAN RUNS ALONGSIDE TRAIN

MOSCOW　　**REUTERS**

A woman whose arm became trapped in a carriage door was forced to run alongside a departing train in central Russia for 400 yards before the driver noticed, a local policeman said.

The police officer, head of a rail police station in the Volga region, said the driver did not immediately see that the woman's arm was trapped in the door of his train at Polivanovo station.

After stopping the train, the driver opened the doors and freed the 35-year-old woman, who was treated in hospital for a gash.

No Sign Of Punishment For Sex At 60 (mph)

BERLIN   REUTERS

Having sex while driving at 60 miles per hour down a highway is not an offense in Germany. But if you hit something make sure you don't run off.

A Cologne court fined a man who admitted he was having sex with a blonde hitchhiker sitting astride him when he drove his car into a road sign. But only because he fled the scene of the accident with his naked accomplice.

"The man was convicted of hit-and-run and sentenced to a fine of 600 euros," a court spokesman said. "It's hard to believe but in fact no law was broken with the intercourse on the motorway. It's a situation lawmakers never thought about."

The 23-year-old man, who was tracked down through the car's registration, was also ordered to pay 400 euros to repair the sign. He did not know the name of the woman who left her clothes behind in the car.

Toddler Crashes Dad's Car Twice In Four Days

BERLIN   REUTERS

A motor-mad three-year-old German boy crashed his father's car twice in four days, police in the western town of Borken said.

Using a ladder, the boy stole the keys to his father's Honda Accord, started the car and plowed it into a nearby Toyota, causing some 5,000 euros ($5,750) of damage but escaping unharmed.

When a television crew came to their home in the town of Bocholt near the Dutch border to reconstruct the incident four days later, the young lad took matters into his own hands.

Sitting behind the wheel with the car key given to him during filming, he was overtaken again by an urge to drive.

"The father was with the television crew," said a Borken police spokesman. "The car was in gear and the boy just started up and drove into the car ahead."

The boy was not hurt, but chalked up further damages totaling around 1,000 euros.

MOTOR-MAD
THREE-
YEAR-OLD

maximum speed
of four miles per
hour

MAN LOSES LICENSE FOR DRIVING LAWN-MOWER DRUNK

BERLIN   REUTERS

A German gardener has been fined and stripped of his license for driving his lawnmower while drunk, a court said.

The court fined the 45-year-old man 400 euros ($460) and banned him from driving all vehicles, including his mower, for three months after police did a check on him as he was parking the vehicle, which has a maximum speed of four miles per hour.

The defense lawyer told Reuters his client would appeal. "The mower does not pose the remotest danger to the public and common sense should have been applied," he said.

Handy Massages At Gas Stations

BANGKOK REUTERS

A massage a day keeps the Thai death toll at bay.

That's the message from Thailand's Health Ministry, which said it planned to set up traditional massage services at gas stations to help motorists relieve stress and, it hoped, cut the road toll.

The ministry, in a statement, said it was working with a Thai fuel company to provide the services in 21 gas stations on major inter-city highways and around the capital Bangkok from next month.

"The more hours people continue to drive on roads, the less concentration motorists tend to have and the more accidents are likely to occur," Vichai Chokevivat, head of the ministry's department of Thai traditional medicine, said in the statement.

"A 15-minute pause for stretching or massage will help relieve their stress," Vichai said.

JOYRIDERS CLOG NEW TRAINS

NEW DELHI   REUTERS

The Indian capital's new $2-billion underground rail system has become such an astonishing success—and headache—since opening, that desperate officials are pleading with customers to stay away.

Built to carry 200,000 passengers a day, it drew more than 1.2 million of Delhi's 13 million people on the first day, most of them simply checking out the city's latest attraction and riding around aimlessly for hours.

The Metro has now run out of electronic tokens after commuters took them as souvenirs and the emergency intercom on the trains has been turned off because passengers were buzzing the driver to tell him to go faster.

Anticipating even heavier demand on the weekend, the Metro management published prominent notices in main newspapers urging people to hold off "pleasure trips."

The high-tech Metro, with air-conditioned, South Korean-made carriages, is the crowded capital's first city rail system and its four rupees (eight U.S. cents) fare makes it affordable even for many poor people.

Man Blames Reckless Driving On Martians

MARSEILLE   REUTERS

A Frenchman who raced through a motorway roadblock, triggering a high-speed police car chase that ended in a minor crash, has blamed aliens from Mars for his reckless driving.

Under police custody in a hospital in the Mediterranean city of Marseille, the 42-year-old told police he was being "chased by Martians" when he charged through a roadblock on the A55 motorway, police sources said.

A breathalyzer test for alcohol proved negative, but police were awaiting the results of drug tests and a psychiatric examination.

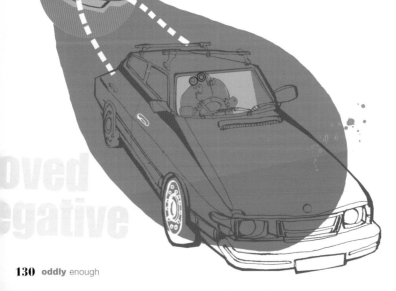

Roadside Sex Romp

TIRANA REUTERS

An amorous Albanian couple's very public highway hanky-panky mortified motorists this week in a country emerging from decades of social conservatism.

The daily *Korrieri* newspaper reported that travelers on an eastern highway were amazed at the cheek of a couple who emerged naked from a car, had a brief roadside romp and then scampered off before the police arrived.

"The couple came out of their car completely naked and started making love on the asphalt," said a taxi driver. "They did not care about onlookers. After a few minutes, they kissed and walked back to their car."

TOURISTS STRAY INTO WAR ZONE

BETHLEHEM | West Bank REUTERS

Two Japanese tourists, eager to visit Bethlehem's Church of the Nativity, were so engrossed in their guide book, they did not notice they had wandered into a war zone.

It was only when news photographers in flak jackets and helmets spotted the oblivious couple and pointed out the bullet-pocked buildings and military hardware around them that they decided to call off their trip to the Christian shrine.

"We have been on the road for the last six months and we did not watch television or read the newspapers," the man told one photographer, who told him the church was the center of an Israeli siege of Palestinian gunmen.

POLICE PULL PLUG ON DRIVE-BY-WIRE CAR

ZURICH   REUTERS

Pull this wire to go faster. Insert plug here for car fan operation.

One Swiss do-it-yourself car repairer was left stranded after Swiss police decided his replacement for a broken accelerator—a wire feeding straight into the engine block—was too innovative to meet road-worthiness standards.

A direct socket and plug connection between the ventilator and car battery also failed to pass their roadside inspection which culminated in the vehicle being impounded.

Kids Take Unwanted Joyride

SYDNEY   REUTERS

A light plane carrying three children but no pilot taxied out of control on a runway in Australia's tropical north and hit three planes parked nearby before it finally came to rest.

None of the children was hurt in the incident at the airport in Darwin, the major city in Australia's vast Northern Territory.

Witnesses said the pilot of the single-engine Cessna 182, owned by the Salvation Army charity group, got out of the plane to crank its propeller by hand.

But the plane moved off before he could get back in and crashed into three stationary small planes before it finally stopped.

Inept Car Thieves Couldn't Drive

EDMONTON | Alberta   REUTERS

Two would-be Canadian thieves learned the hard way on New Year's Day that knowing how to drive a car is a prerequisite for stealing one.

Police said the two males accosted a pizza deliveryman in northeast Edmonton, Alberta, and demanded the four pizzas he was carrying as well as cash.

The bandits, aged 17 and 18, apparently changed their minds at one point and jumped into the man's car.

But their getaway was foiled because the 17-year-old behind the wheel did not know how to drive a stick shift.

Flummoxed by the manual transmission and clutch, the duo then went back to their original plan to commandeer the pizzas, an Edmonton police spokesman said.

"It was a toss-up between pizzas and the car, and they knew how to operate pizzas," he added.

FAKE SQUEEGEE KIDS NAB SCOFFLAWS

VANCOUVER | British Columbia   REUTERS

Drivers in Burnaby, British Columbia, should make sure they are buckled up the next time a "squeegee kid" approaches offering to wash their windshield.

Royal Canadian Mounted Police in the Vancouver suburb have been posing as the car window washers at major intersections in a bid to catch people who are breaking the law by not wearing seat belts when they drive.

In a four-hour period this week, officers issued 90 tickets. "It's been very successful," Constable Phil Reid said.

The undercover officer washing the window looks inside the car to see if the seat belts are properly attached. If not, they give a quiet signal, and a uniformed officer a short distance down the road stops the car again.

"If you're lucky, you just get your windshield cleaned," Reid said.

It is actually illegal to offer street window washing in Burnaby, but Reid said police were allowed to break some laws as part of the undercover operation.

Three Times Unlucky For Driver

STOCKHOLM REUTERS

Swedish police caught a drunk Norwegian driver three times in as many hours on the weekend, a Swedish newspaper reported.

Police pulled the man over after spotting him hitting speeds of 85 miles per hour, double the normal speed limit, the daily *Aftonbladet* said.

Officers found he had an alcohol level of more than three times the maximum allowed under Swedish law.

Police confiscated the man's driver's license but set him free.

Undeterred, he drove on toward Norway but was caught, and released, a second time.

The Norwegian tried his luck a third time but was caught yet again, and this time a prosecutor confiscated his car.

TRIED HIS LUCK A THI

SEEING BELFAST—
TANKS FOR THE TOUR

BELFAST   REUTERS

Tourists wanting to take in the hot spots of Belfast now have a safe way to do so.

A pair of entrepreneurs from Northern Ireland's capital, famous worldwide for its sectarian troubles, have bought two half-century-old British military armored cars to drive tourists around.

"We found them on the Internet," one of the pair, Art Corbett, told Reuters. "Tourists love it, it's pandemonium!"

Although they were brought over from Britain, the Humber Pig and Saladin vehicles both served in Northern Ireland during the three-decade "Troubles" in which more than 3,000 people were killed. Despite running on wheels, they are thick-plated and called "tanks" by Belfast people.

While the 1998 Good Friday agreement has not ended violence altogether in the British-ruled province, it has paved the way for a mini-tourism boom.

These Air Traffic Controllers Are Getting Younger All The Time...

LONDON   REUTERS

Instead of landing instructions, pilots in aircraft approaching Britain's Luton airport heard the squealing of a tiny infant broadcast over their radios.

Authorities worked 12 hours to track the frequency and determined that a baby monitor at the mother's house, located near the airport, was broadcasting her baby's cries to the cockpits of approaching planes, the BBC reported.

"It was like something out of the Ghostbusters. They came down the path and stopped me and said we'd like to check something inside the house," the mother told the station.

The BBC said there was no threat to safety; pilots who heard the infant instead of air traffic control were able to switch to a different frequency.

The company that made the baby monitor supplied the family with a new one.

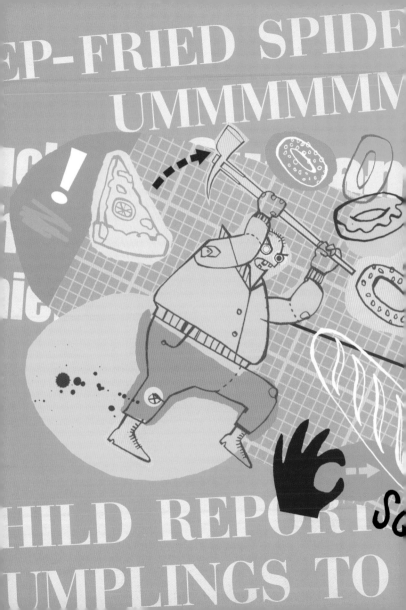

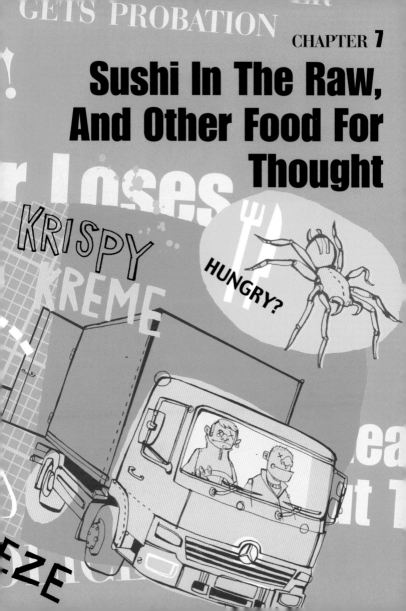

Stolen Truck Leaves Long Doughnut Trail

SLIDELL | LA   REUTERS

Two people left a 15-mile-long trail of doughnuts after they took a Krispy Kreme truck from a parking lot and fled, police said.

The truck was parked at a convenience store with its rear doors open and engine running while a deliveryman carried doughnuts inside, said a Slidell police spokesman.

Two suspects hopped in the truck and sped off to the nearby town of Lacombe with doughnuts spilling out along the way, he said.

They abandoned the truck when they were spotted by police responding to reports of a dangerous driver who was losing his doughnuts. A passenger was captured, but the driver, whose name was not released, ran away.

The passenger, a woman, told police they had been smoking crack cocaine for several hours before the incident, the spokesman said.

Their motive for taking the Krispy Kreme truck was unclear.

"I don't know if it was a need for transportation or if they just had the munchies," he said.

"…THEY JUST HAD THE MUNCHIES"

TASTY, IF YOU LIKE POISON

ABBOTSFORD | British Columbia REUTERS

A Canadian nursery scrambled to locate the final missing shipments of a poisonous plant accidentally sent to stores with labels that said they were "tasty in soup."

An employee playing a "stupid joke" led to the dangerously incorrect labels being applied to pots of Autumn Monkshood shipped to stores in Ontario, Idaho, Washington state and British Columbia, according to the nursery.

Autumn Monkshood, a perennial plant with violet-blue flowers, is poisonous even when cooked, but the labels attached to the pots said: "All parts of this plant are tasty in soup," according to the company.

Eating the plants could cause paralysis of the heart.

A nursery employee crossed out "poisonous" on a proof-sheet of the labels—mistakenly thinking the sheets would be checked by a horticultural expert before going to the printer—and put them on the pots, a company official told Reuters.

Customer Loses Appetite Over Toilets

STOCKHOLM   REUTERS

A customer in an international hamburger chain outlet in western Sweden lost his appetite when he discovered the restaurant's toilet seats were being washed in its dishwasher alongside the kitchen utensils.

The man noticed on a visit to the bathroom in the restaurant in Arvika, Sweden, that all the toilet seats had been removed.

When he asked staff about the missing seats, an employee took them out of a dishwasher where they had been cleaned together with trays and kitchen utensils, the Swedish TT news agency reported, quoting the regional newspaper *Nya Wermlands-Tidningen*.

The employee tried to reassure the customer by saying that the freshly washed toilet seat would be warm and pleasant to sit on.

A senior representative of the restaurant chain said the incident was a mistake and not standard company procedure. Arvika's environmental and health inspector later visited the restaurant.

TOILET SEATS HAD BEEN REMOVED

Round Of "Firewater" Leaves Drinkers With Burns

VIENNA   REUTERS

A round of "schnapps" on the house landed an Austrian waiter and his customers in the hospital after he served them dishwasher fluid that left them with internal burns.

After knocking back the shots in a bar in the southern town of Klagenfurt, the four drinkers were seized by coughing fits and their eyes turned watery and red, police said.

They complained to the waiter, who then downed a glass himself and also began coughing.

The five were rushed to a hospital where they were treated for burns to the mouth and gullet.

Police said the accident happened after a bartender had decided to refill the schnapps bottle with washing detergent.

CHILD REPORTS DUMPLINGS TO POLICE

LINZ | Austria   REUTERS

A four-year-old Austrian boy was so disgusted by his grandmother's plum dumplings that he dialed emergency services for help, Austrian state television ORF said.

When the startled policeman on the other end of the line in Linz asked the young caller what he thought the police should do, the boy was clueless, the report said.

The officer pleaded with the boy to give grandmother's plum dumplings another chance. He agreed and hung up.

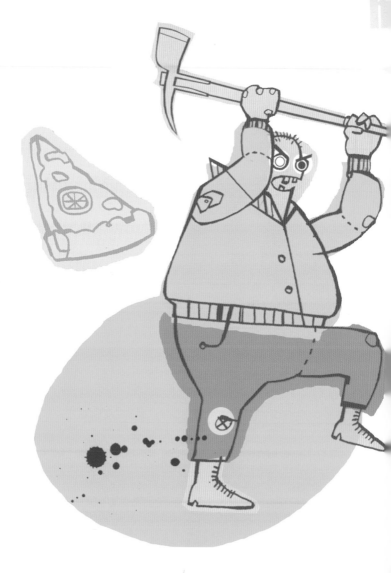

AXEMAN ATTACKS CHEF OVER PIZZA

FRANKFURT　　REUTERS

Unhappy with his pizza and not content with a refund, a man in Germany has gone after the chef with an axe.

Frankfurt police said the 57-year-old man was restrained by customers after he drew the axe from his coat and started swinging it at the cook.

"Apparently, the pizza didn't agree with him," said a police spokesman. "He wasn't a regular customer."

The drunken man, who had been offered a refund or a fresh pizza after complaining his first one was revolting, was ejected from the restaurant after shouting abuse.

He later returned to continue his tirade and then produced the axe and attempted to strike the chef but patrons managed to wrestle him to the ground. He was arrested by police.

"COOKIE CRUMBLER" GETS PROBATION

PHILADELPHIA · REUTERS

His deeds may not rise to the infamy of the Joker, the Riddler or the Penguin. But as the "Cookie Crumbler," he won his own place in the annals of crime.

The 38-year-old advertising executive, convicted of squeezing, poking and crumbling baked goods valued at $1,000 during criminally finicky shopping sprees in suburban Philadelphia, was sentenced this week to 180 days' probation—90 days each for the bread and the cookies.

He was also ordered to pay $1,000 in restitution.

"You engaged in behavior that was not just odd, it was criminal," the *Philadelphia Inquirer* quoted the judge as telling the man at a sentencing hearing. "You caused harm to people."

Sensationalized as the "Cookie Crumbler" by local news outlets, the man was accused of manhandling bread and cookies at suburban supermarkets over a two-year period that ended in 1999, when he moved to Las Vegas.

Police charged him with two counts of criminal mischief. He denied wrongdoing at his trial, even though footage from in-store surveillance cameras showed him poking and prodding boxes of cookies and running his hands over dozens of loaves of bread.

Two bakeries claimed that the man caused irreparable damage to products valued at nearly $8,000. His wife testified at trial that he was simply a picky shopper who wanted to ensure freshness for his family.

" ...not just odd, it was criminal"

Ad Backfires Over Cyanide Fears

LONDON REUTERS

The makers of an Italian liqueur have pulled a novel advertising campaign involving wafting the scent of almonds around London Underground stations, after fears that the sweet aroma might be confused with cyanide.

The 1.5 million pound ($2.4 million) plan used metal boxes full of almond oils which were positioned at the bottom of escalators in three major stations.

Fans in each box spread the scent around with the idea of prompting travelers to associate it with the aroma of Di Saronno amaretto liqueur.

Advertising posters all the way up the side wall of the escalators aimed to help them make the connection.

Unfortunately, as amateur sleuths and readers of Agatha Christie know, almonds smell like cyanide—not a great selling point at a time of heightened terrorist alert.

Only three days after the scheme began, the British distributors of the drink withdrew it.

We Always Suspected They Did This...

BERLIN REUTERS

A German judge fined an ill-tempered pizza delivery man $610 for spitting into a salad order, a court said.

The court said the 32-year-old man was angry because he had to make an extra delivery to a couple who complained they had not received their salad. After discovering a globule of saliva under a slice of cucumber, the pair informed local police.

Laboratory tests conducted on the pizza delivery courier's saliva established his culpability.

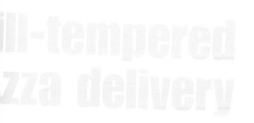

ill-tempered
zza delivery

DEEP-FRIED SPIDER! UMMMMMMM!

SKUON | Cambodia   REUTERS

First unearthed by starving Cambodians in the dark days of the Khmer Rouge "killing fields" rule, Skuon's spiders have transformed from the vital sustenance of desperate refugees into a choice national delicacy.

Black, hairy and packing vicious, venom-soaked fangs, the burrowing arachnids common to the jungle around this bustling market town do not appear at first sight to be the caviar of Cambodia.

But for many residents of Skuon, the "a-ping"—as the breed of palm-sized tarantula is known in Khmer—are a source of fame and fortune in an otherwise impoverished farming region in the east of the war-ravaged southeast Asian nation.

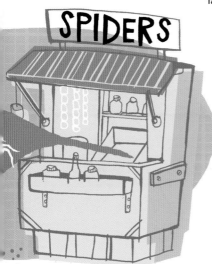

"On a good day, I can sell between 100 and 200 spiders," said a spider seller who supports her entire family by hawking the creepy-crawlies, deep fried in garlic and salt, to the people who flock to Skuon for a juicy morsel.

SALAMI "GUN" CAUSES POLICE ALERT

BERLIN   REUTERS

A man who mistook salami for an automatic pistol triggered a major police operation in southern Germany involving 10 police cars and a helicopter.

The man alerted police that he had seen three men handling a gun in a car at a motorway service area. Police cars, dogs and a helicopter chased the car and held up the men, only to identify the "weapon" as a salami.

"Behind the dirty windows of the car, the man had mistaken the salami for a gun," a police spokesman in Traunstein said. "The men in the car had probably passed the sausage through the car."

The salami was returned to its owners, he said.

Luck Runs Out For Chocolate Cake Thief

MEXICO CITY REUTERS

It was a tasty heist while it lasted.

For four straight mornings, a thief with a sweet tooth rushed into a pastry shop in Mexico City and held up the duty employee at knifepoint before making off with a chocolate cake.

His mistake, however, was to pounce every day at 8 a.m. sharp. So, the Azteca pastry shop's manager called in the police a few minutes ahead of time and they nabbed the thief as he tried to pull off the cake heist for a fifth straight day.

"He arrived at the pastry shop armed with a knife and again demanded his cake from the employee, but when he tried to escape he was arrested by the police," Mexico City's police department said in a statement.

It said the thief and the chocolate cake were then both handed over to judicial authorities.

Store Seeks Dedicated Chocoholic

LONDON   REUTERS

Calling all chocoholics. One of Britain's most exclusive grocery stores needs a new chocolate taster—and will pay 35,000 pounds ($54,400) a year for the successful candidate.

Fortnum & Mason in London's Piccadilly—one of the capital's most prestigious addresses—is looking for a chocolate buyer to travel the world, taste as much chocolate as possible, and select only the best for its discerning customers.

The *Daily Telegraph* newspaper said Fortnum's personnel director had already been bombarded with applications after she advertised the post as the "best job in the world."

But not all of those interested had the right qualifications.

"We only advertised it on Sunday," she told the *Telegraph*. "But already we have had loads of people writing in saying they have absolutely no experience, or they work in the metal industry or something, but they love chocolate."

GOURMET BURGLARS FEAST IN RESTAURANTS

VIENNA   REUTERS

Gourmet burglars have targeted restaurants in northern Austria, leaving behind empty cash registers—and a pile of dirty dishes.

"That is just so cheeky, they plundered my supplies," said one restaurateur, after burglars raided the till and then had a beer and a bite in his kitchen.

"They ate a whole kilo of bread and my best sausages," the restaurateur was quoted as saying in the Austrian tabloid *Kronen*.

The daily mentioned similar cases, also in the province of Lower Austria, where thieves cooked up steaks in the kitchens after emptying restaurants of cash.

HIS BEER HAS THEM SPINNING

BERLIN — REUTERS

A German priest has developed a novel way to brew beer—in a washing machine.

The priest, from the western city of Duisburg, came up with the idea of converting his 35-year-old toploader to provide beer more cheaply for youth outings he organizes.

"All I needed was something that could be used to heat and stir the mix—so why not a washing machine?" said the priest, who now uses another machine for his clothes.

His machine brews 40 pints of beer in 10 hours.

The priest said his unorthodox brewing method had made him consider experimenting with new flavors: "I recently read about some American beer made with chilies. Now that could be interesting."

UNORTHODOX
BREWING METHODS

Pitch Dark Bar For Blind Dates

BERLIN   REUTERS

Diners at Berlin's newest restaurant cannot see their meal and are guided to their table by blind waiters because the bar is pitch black.

The restaurant aims to make guests concentrate on senses other than sight. Holding on to one another, the first visitors followed their waiter into the dining room. Although the PhD student has been blind since childhood, he is the only one able to point out chairs, cutlery, and drinks.

"I'm putting your plate right in front of you," the waiter said.

"I can't find my mouth," one voice replied out of the dark. "I wonder what this dish is—lasagna? Or some casserole?" another invisible guest pondered out loud.

In the "unsicht-Bar," which means invisible in German, diners cannot choose complete dishes from the menu as they would normally do. Instead, they can only indicate whether they would like a fish, meat or vegetarian option.

"We want people to have an extraordinary experience of tasting, feeling, and smelling," said the head of the organization for blind and sight-restricted people, which is running the bar.

"People are surprised that their tongues and taste senses are taking over and are sending signals, which their eyes would normally have sent," he added.

Of the 30 staff, 22 are blind.

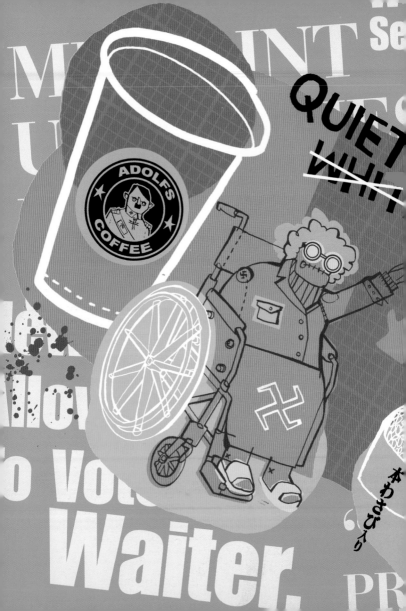

Hunchbacks, Hitler And More Sensitive Topics

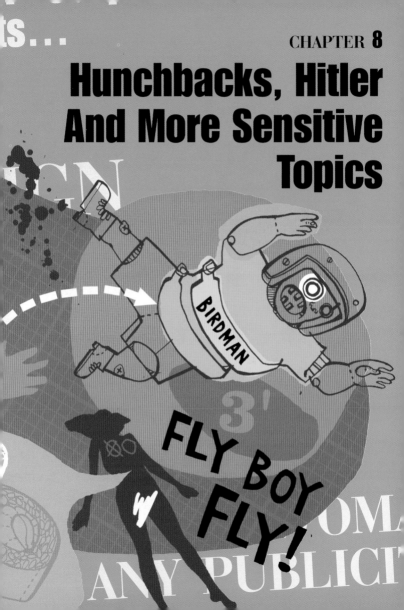

MISPRINT UNLEASHES HATE CAMPAIGN ON LANDLADY

LONDON   REUTERS

A British seaside landlady was targeted by a hate campaign after an advertisement for an apartment flat mistakenly said she was seeking a "white person" as a tenant rather than a "quiet person," newspapers reported.

The woman, a disabled grandmother who used to be a nurse, insisted she was no racist and the advertisement was a misprint by a local newspaper in the coastal town of Brighton.

She was inundated by protest calls, while a local pressure group issued a statement demanding the police investigate her under the Race Discrimination Act, said Britain's *Daily Telegraph* newspaper.

"Lots of people have rung up over the weekend swearing at me... I've tried to explain, but they don't listen," she was quoted as saying. "I'm now frightened to pick up the phone."

"I sponsor a nine-year-old girl in Zimbabwe called Becky," she added. "I would hardly do something like that if I was prejudiced."

Political Correctness Rings Hunchback Death Knell

LONDON REUTERS

A British theater company has dropped the word hunchback from its stage adaptation of the classic novel "The Hunchback of Notre Dame" to avoid offending disabled people, newspapers reported.

Oddsocks Productions has renamed its touring production "The Bellringer of Notre Dame" after discussions with a disability adviser raised the possibility of offending people with spina bifida or the disfiguring scoliosis of the spine.

"We have not changed the novel in any way, we simply felt changing the title would cause less offense," the producer was quoted as saying by the *Daily Mirror*.

He May Be Wascally, But He's Not A Sexist

OTTAWA   REUTERS

Bugs Bunny may be a wascally hare-brained rabbit, but at least he's not a sexist one.

The Canadian Broadcasting Standards Council said it had rejected a complaint from an angry woman who accused the cartoon character of having made a deeply misogynistic comment.

The incident was triggered by an episode of the "Bugs Bunny and Tweety" show aired in July 1998. It featured a short cartoon entitled "Bewitched Bunny" in which Bugs escaped a witch by detonating a bag of so-called magic powder.

A beautiful female rabbit emerged from the cloud of dust and took Bugs by the arm. As the two of them walked off into the sunset, Bugs turned to the camera and said: "Ah sure, I know! But aren't they all witches inside?"

Kapow! One woman watching the show on Canada's Global Television was less than amused and fired off a letter to the channel's president.

Global replied that the cartoon in fact portrayed the female characters in a strong light.

"SKANK" NOT LIBEL, APPEALS COURT RULES

SAN FRANCISCO　　REUTERS

It may not be great to be a skank but legally it is okay to be called one.

A California state appeals court has ruled it is not libel to call someone a "skank" or even a "big skank" on the radio—describing the word as "a derogatory slang term of recent vintage that has no generally recognized meaning."

The state's 1st Court of Appeals, ruling in a case stemming from the Fox special "Who Wants to Marry a Multimillionaire," found that participants in the program "voluntarily subjected themselves to inevitable scrutiny and potential ridicule by the public and the media."

A contestant, one of 50 women who competed to marry a multimillionaire on the highly rated show, sued two morning disc jockeys at a San Francisco radio station after they called her a "local loser," a "chicken-butt," and a "skank" for declining their invitation to appear on their show.

The woman was not amused and sued the disc jockeys, their producer and the radio station owner, accusing them of slander, invasion of privacy and infliction of emotional distress.

But the appeals court judges, in their ruling, instructed the trial court to dismiss the case, saying the on-air discussion involved "a television show of significant interest to the public and the media" and thus was a protected form of free speech.

The appeals court also rejected the plaintiff's claim that she was libeled, saying there was no way to prove that the disc jockeys had knowingly perpetrated a falsehood by describing her as a "local loser," a "chicken butt," and a "big skank."

"big skank"

"TALENTLESS" WOMAN PROVES ANY PUBLICITY IS GOOD

STOCKHOLM REUTERS

Negative advertising works, at least for a Swedish care worker who gave it a try after fruitless attempts to find a new job by more conventional means.

"I want a well-paid job. I have no imagination, I am anti-social, uncreative, and untalented," read an advertisement posted by the 30-year-old woman.

Her phone started ringing incessantly and job offers poured in, she said.

"I turned everything upside down. I was so tired to do things the ordinary way," she told the Internet edition of the daily *Expressen*.

She has an interview on Wednesday with a company offering an increase of more than 30 percent over her present salary, she said.

Waiter, There's A Naked Lady In My Sushi

BONN REUTERS

A German restaurant has been attacked as "tasteless" for serving sushi on naked models lying on top of tables.

An ombudsman for women's issues in the central city of Hanover said she was appalled that the restaurant saw nothing wrong with using naked women as huge "platters" for the Japanese dish, dubbed "sushi ala Jungfrau (virgin)."

But the restaurant owner was quoted by *Bild* newspaper as saying the dish had been a huge hit and the evening-long meal, costing up to 400 marks ($250) per person, was booked out for weeks in advance.

The models, usually students in their 20s, wear nothing but see-through veils over their heads and a thin floral decoration between their legs. They are required to lie motionless on the table in the extra warm room.

The sushi is spread out all over their bodies. Bodyguards dressed as samurai warriors make sure nothing gets out of hand.

"They aren't entirely naked," wrote *Bild*. "Caviar is stuffed into their belly buttons, sword fish sushi is stuck near their armpits and between their legs is raw tuna fish sushi awaiting the hungry guests."

本わさび入り

PUNCH AND JUDY GET A POUNDING

LONDON REUTERS

A local British council may ban Punch and Judy puppet shows in case the traditional Italian slugfest disturbs children.

Punch and Judy shows have occupied a hallowed place in British entertainment since the 17th century, with children gleefully hollering at the hump-backed, hook-nosed Mr Punch as he relentlessly wields a stick on his put-upon wife Judy.

But Colchester borough council in Essex, southern England, says that the wife beating seen in a typical Punch and Judy show is no laughing matter in an era where we all too often see broken homes, domestic violence and political correctness.

"Young children are very impressionable. Seeds are sown at a very young age," the head of the council's art and leisure committee told BBC radio.

She conceded there wouldn't be much left if the blows had to go, but said the council might still issue its ban.

Puppet masters insist the age-old show is fun, moral and arty, firmly in the tradition of Italy's *commedia dell'arte*.

"Mr Punch's weapon is, of course, the slapstick—a pantomime weapon making a great noise with the pretence of dealing a heavy blow," said the coordinator of the Punch and Judy College of Professors. "We're not actually talking about real violence here. We're talking about knockabout comedy. The same comedy that Tom and Jerry engage in."

Muslim Woman Must Drop Veil For License

MIAMI REUTERS

A Muslim woman who cited religious reasons in refusing to remove her veil for a driver's license photo must show her face for the camera if she wants her license reinstated, a Florida judge ruled.

In a case that pitted claims of religious freedom against security concerns, a judge ruled that Florida has a compelling interest in identifying drivers during traffic stops and that photo images are essential to promote that interest.

"The requirement that all potential drivers have their driver's license photos taken unveiled, uncloaked and unmasked does not unconstitutionally burden the free exercise of religion," the judge wrote.

The plaintiff obtained a Florida driver's license that showed her wearing a black veil with only her eyes uncovered in February 2001. Seven months later, the Florida Department of Highway Safety and Motor Vehicles notified her that her license would be revoked unless she was photographed with her face showing.

SECURITY CONCERNS

New Law Allows Drunks To Vote

OSLO REUTERS

It will be two pints of lager and a ballot, please, in Norway this year after a change in the law allowing voters to get drunk and then go out to vote.

"The election board can no longer refuse anyone to vote because they are intoxicated," an adviser at the Local Government Ministry said.

Until recently, Norway's election law has denied entry to polling stations to anyone with "seriously impaired judgment" or "reduced consciousness" from booze, but that law has been scrapped, adviser Steinar Dalbakk told the *Bladet Tromsoe* newspaper.

But Norwegians will have to sober up again for the 2005 general elections. Politicians—possibly fearing the effects of a political hangover—have re-enacted the law banning drunken voting.

TENANTS SOUGHT FOR "HAUNTED" APARTMENTS

HONG KONG   REUTERS

The Hong Kong Housing Authority is looking for people to rent 77 apartments widely believed to be haunted, the *South China Morning Post* reported.

Gruesome murders and suicides have taken place in some of the apartments, which are among 3,000 units with "unfavorable conditions" being offered to help needy families find affordable housing, the newspaper reported.

The units could bring a total of at least HK$3 million (US$384,600) per month for the Housing Authority, if there are takers.

Ghosts aside, "unfavorable conditions" also refer to apartments close to rubbish dumps and those with common bathrooms and kitchens.

Even though property prices have plunged 50–60 percent from their 1997 peaks, Hong Kong remains one of the most expensive cities in the world.

About 10,000 applicants are expected to apply for the units, all of which are immediately available.

BLACK CHURCH OFFERS MONEY TO LURE WHITES

NEW ORLEANS | LA   REUTERS

A black Baptist minister looking to diversify his church wants to pay white people to attend his sermons.

For the month of August, whites who go to Greenwood Acres Full Gospel Baptist Church in Shreveport, Louisiana, will get $5 an hour on Sundays and $10 an hour on Thursdays, Bishop Fred Caldwell told Reuters.

Caldwell said his 5,000-member church has been almost exclusively black since it was founded in 1958, which he thinks was not the way Jesus wanted it.

"The most segregated hour in America, depending on the time zone, is 11 o'clock Sunday morning," he said.

Caldwell first announced the offer in his sermon on Sunday, telling the congregation the money would come out of his own pocket, not church coffers. Supportive members have offered to help pay.

So far, he said, the church has gotten more than 100 phone calls from whites wanting to attend, with many offering to forgo the money. The motives of those who want the cash are not questioned, Caldwell said.

"Jesus said that we're to fish for men," he said. "I'm just using money to fish with."

Caldwell said his budget is limited to several thousand dollars and for now the offer will go only to whites. Hispanics, Asians, and other ethnic groups will have to wait.

"I'm only paying for white folks in August," Caldwell said. "We'll probably move on to other ethnic groups from there."

Well, All Couples Have Some Secrets...

COLOMBO REUTERS

A young Sri Lankan woman has filed for divorce three months into her marriage after discovering her husband was really a woman, a newspaper reported.

The young bride had been whisked away on her wedding night by her parents who were suspicious about the groom's feminine gait and high-pitched voice, the *Daily Mirror* reported.

The matter ended up in a court in the capital Colombo when the transvestite groom "had gone to the girl's residence to take his wife back," the paper said.

The paper did not say how the bride was lured into the marriage but said the transvestite had carried out similar scams in the past.

Ban On "Dwarf Throwing" Upheld

GENEVA   REUTERS

A tiny stuntman who protested a French ban on the bizarre practice of "dwarf throwing" lost his case before a U.N. human rights body which said the need to protect human dignity was paramount.

The man had argued the 1995 ban by France's highest administrative court was discriminatory and deprived him of a job being hurled around discotheques by burly men.

In a statement the U.N. Human Rights Committee said it was satisfied "the ban on dwarf-tossing was not abusive but necessary in order to protect public order, including considerations of human dignity." The committee also said the ban "did not amount to prohibited discrimination."

The pastime, imported from the United States and Australia in the 1980s, consists of people throwing tiny stuntmen as far as they possibly can, usually in a bar or discotheque.

The stuntman wears a crash helmet and padded clothing which has handles on the back to facilitate throwing the human projectile.

The Frenchman, who measures 3 feet 10 inches tall, filed his case in 1999 with the U.N. committee made up of 18 independent experts who examine states' compliance with the 1976 International Covenant on Civil and Political Rights.

"FREAK SHOW" JOB AD ENRAGES RIGHTS GROUP

PERTH   REUTERS

A job advertisement seeking human "freaks" including a bearded woman and a rubber person for a 19th century-style sideshow has upset human rights campaigners in Australia.

Corporate Theatre Productions, a theatrical production company, has received six replies to the advertisement it first ran in the state of Western Australia, the manager said.

He said he was looking for professional performers to be part of a sideshow to entertain people at an exhibition of plumbing hardware in Perth.

"The aim is to recreate the atmosphere of a Barnum and Bailey circus," he said.

TOSSING

DRAG QUEEN MAKE-UP COURSE

MELBOURNE REUTERS

An Australian college has introduced a drag queen make-up course to meet rising demand for the skill to hide beard shadows and to enter the glitzy glamour of the drag world.

The course, targeted at occasional drag queens, cross dressers and make-up students, has also sparked wider interest from those who want to know the basics about the thick, theatrical style make-up.

"Even the quietest, shiest person really comes to life," the lecturer told Reuters.

"It is a way of transforming yourself. I think there is a suppressed performer in everybody."

Students will have the opportunity to don wigs and their favorite dresses at the end of the make-up course as they take on their complete drag queen persona.

occasional drag queens

Waiter Gets Revenge Over Veggie Order

LOS ANGELES   REUTERS

Sometimes, a waiter just gets one complaint too many.

Police in Corona, California, say a waiter at a restaurant there went to the home of a family who complained about his service and cooked up a special order on their lawn—eggs, flour, maple syrup, and toilet paper.

The 20-year-old waiter was arrested on suspicion of vandalism and contributing to the delinquency of minors—his 17-year-old girlfriend and two younger brothers—who helped him deliver the midnight snack, police said.

A spokeswoman for the restaurant said the waiter had been fired.

The waiter apparently became incensed when a customer complained to a manager that he refused to swap the potatoes that came with her meal for vegetables.

After throwing eggs against the customer's house, festooning the trees with toilet paper and sprinkling the lawn with flour and maple syrup, the waiter and his crew rang the doorbell several times around 1 a.m. and waited to see the reaction, police said.

Have We Got A Job For You!

BERLIN   REUTERS

A Berlin job center unwittingly offered an unemployed woman work in a brothel.

"The advert just said they were looking for someone to work in a massage parlor. We weren't to know it was a brothel," said a spokesman for the government-run agency in Berlin's central Mitte district.

"It is a bit embarrassing though," he said.

Rage rather than embarrassment was the response of the 25-year-old woman, who has been looking for work without success in Germany's cash-strapped capital.

"It really is a bit much if the job center assumes that the best thing is for you to try your luck in a whorehouse," she told *Tageszeitung* newspaper.

"We'll spoil you with hot kisses, tender and loving massages or no-holds-barred sex," the brothel says of its employees on its Web site.

COFFEE SHOP CHAIN APOLOGIZES FOR HITLER QUOTE

HONG KONG   REUTERS

Popular Hong Kong coffee shop chain Pacific Coffee publicly apologized for carrying in its shops a "thought for the day" by Nazi dictator Adolf Hitler which some customers found offensive.

The quote—"The victor will never be asked if he told the truth"—was chalked on blackboards above the counters in some of its coffee shops.

"I wish to apologize unreservedly, both personally and on behalf of Pacific Coffee Company, for the extremely unfortunate quote that recently appeared on our 'thought for the day' blackboards," the managing director said in a quarter-page advertisement in the front section of the *South China Morning Post*.

"It was morally offensive and inexcusable, and we have instituted controls to ensure that an event like this cannot occur again," it said.

"...morrally offensive and inexcusable"

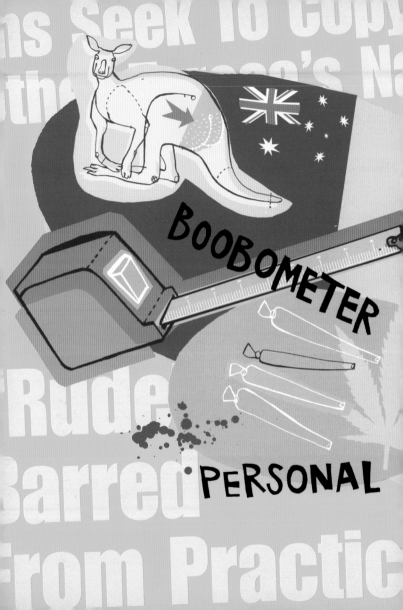

CHAPTER 9

ODD Law: Justice Loses Its Appeal?

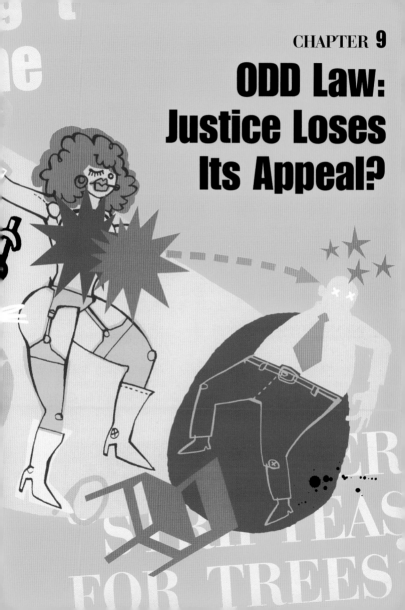

MAN GUILTY OF "GROSS INGRATITUDE"

BERLIN   REUTERS

A German court found a man guilty of "gross ingratitude" and ordered him to pay back a gift of $21,000 after telling his wife she was insane.

A court in the southern town of Coburg ruled that by repeatedly saying she was "crazy and belonged in the funny farm," the man forfeited the right to keep the money she had given him as a present earlier in their marriage.

The couple has since separated. The man refused to return the money and told the court he was provoked by his wife in a series of heated rows. The relationship deteriorated as the couple's business began to struggle.

"Anyone who threatens their partner with the veiled threat of institutionalization is unfit for a present of this size," the court said in its ruling.

Man Sues After Finding Girl Not His Daughter

MELBOURNE   REUTERS

An Australian man is suing his former partner to recover more than $10,000 he spent on a little girl for such things as presents, zoo trips and meals after discovering she was not his daughter, a newspaper said.

"I want it all back—every cent for every toy, every blanket, every bit of food," said the man, who couldn't be identified for legal reasons.

"I wouldn't have spent all that money had I known five years ago she wasn't my kid," he was quoted as saying by the *Herald-Sun*.

The claims include take-away McDonald's food over five years, four visits to an amusement park, three Barbie dolls, a Pooh Bear play tent, a day of skating and child support payments.

The *Herald-Sun* said the man took the action after DNA tests found the girl was not his daughter.

The girl's mother said she was willing to repay the child support payments but that she should not have to pay back anything else.

"She had a good time with him. That's the main thing," she was quoted as saying. "I don't think he should carry on too much about it. He should treat it like doing something nice with a friend."

Nuns Seek To Copyright Mother Teresa's Name

CALCUTTA | India   REUTERS

The order of nuns founded by Mother Teresa seeks to copyright her name in a bid to stop other organizations—from banks to business schools—trying to cash in on the Nobel peace laureate's image worldwide.

"We are seeking legal protection for the use of our logo, and also want such protection for the name of Mother Teresa and that of the Missionaries of Charity," the head of the order said in a statement.

The Missionaries of Charity, established in 1950, says it has received reports that several organizations are using Mother Teresa's name as well as the order's logo—a cross set within an oval and surrounded by rosary beads.

In one case, the order managed to convince the "Mother Teresa Institute of Management" to drop the name. Media reports said a bank was among other organizations trying to capitalize on the name.

The Missionaries of Charity

COURT ORDERS BROTHEL TO REFUND SEX BILL

BERLIN   REUTERS

A German court has ordered a brothel to reimburse a man charged for sex he could not remember having— after the establishment failed to provide an itemized receipt for services rendered.

"The brothel failed to provide concrete documentation of the prices and services provided," said a court spokeswoman in Duesseldorf.

"They should have, for example, listed two sexual intercourse sessions at 600 euros, oral sex at 300 euros or anal sex at 400 euros a go," she told Reuters.

The man told the court he had been too drunk to remember what sexual services he may have ordered at the brothel in Kaarst. The establishment charged him 9,000 euros on his credit card. The brothel owner testified he had ordered the "full program."

Man Claims Injury By Dancer's Breasts

TAMPA | **Fla.**   REUTERS

A Florida man has filed suit against a nightclub, claiming he suffered whiplash when a topless dancer knocked him out with her oversized breasts, the *Tampa Tribune* reported.

"Apparently she jumped up and slammed her breasts on my head and just about knocked me out," the newspaper quoted the plaintiff as saying. "It was like two cement blocks hit me. I saw stars. I've never been right since."

The 38-year-old man filed suit in Pinellas County Court seeking more than $15,000 in damages from the Diamond Dolls club. The dancer, known as Tawny Peaks, was not named in the lawsuit.

According to the lawsuit, the man and friends visited the bar on Sept. 27, 1996, for his bachelor party. Because he was the guest of honor, the dancers asked him to sit on a low chair, rest his head on the back of the chair and close his eyes.

The lawsuit said Peaks danced in front of him and without warning or consent "jumped on the plaintiff forcing her very large breasts into his face causing his head to jerk backward."

The man suffered head, neck and other injuries that caused bodily injury, disability, pain and suffering, disfigurement, mental anguish, and loss of capacity for the enjoyment of life, the suit said.

"It was like two cement blocks hit me."

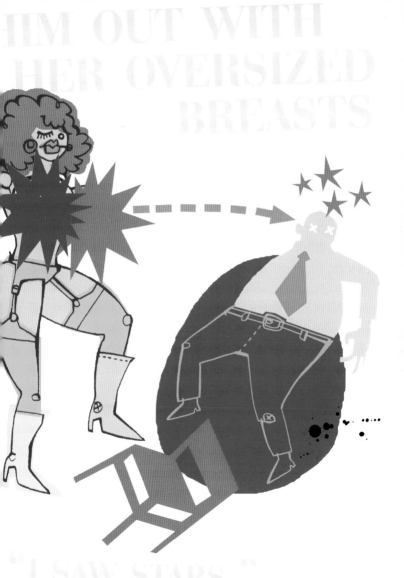

"I SAW STARS."

PROTESTERS "STRIPTEASE FOR TREES"

EUREKA | Calif   REUTERS

Nine bare-breasted women briefly halted logging work near California's contested Headwaters Forest in a protest against what they said was unconscionable logging of redwood trees.

"These gorgeous young women were belly dancing. One logger actually got down on his knees and kissed the ground," said a California activist who has staged several "Strip Tease for the Trees" protests.

She said the protest interrupted logging work for about two hours at a point known as the "Hole in the Headwaters," an area of second-growth redwood trees left out of a 1999 deal between Pacific Lumber Inc. and state and federal officials aimed at preserving the Headwaters Forest about 250 miles north of San Francisco.

The protesters, who gathered around 5 a.m., stripped off their shirts, sang, chanted, and handed out chocolates to surprised loggers, tying up traffic for about two hours until police arrived to clear up the scene. There were no arrests.

"The loggers and the cops were absolutely stunned," said the activist, who launched her anti-logging protests last year with demonstrations of what she calls "goddess-based, nude Buddhist guerrilla poetry" at a number of timber and logging sites in and around northern California.

The action marked the largest environmental striptease to date.

One of the protesters, a 22-year-old, said she was surprised at how agreeable the loggers were when confronted by topless women.

"Rude" Doctor Barred From Practice

LONDON   REUTERS

A British surgeon reported to have told a patient "you have cancer, I have asthma, we all have to die some time" was struck off the rolls.

The General Medical Council said the doctor's conduct "has rightly been described as bizarre."

The surgeon, dubbed "a walking terror in a white coat" by the media, made lewd remarks to female colleagues and occasionally groped them. He wrote nasty and deliberately misleading references about junior doctors, the GMC said.

He also sent a flirtatious card to a young female patient trying to arrange a date without her parents finding out.

And he had a habit of informing patients they had cancer in a manner that was "abrupt, insensitive, rude and below a reasonable professional standard," the council found.

He once informed a patient who had been told she may have gallstones "words to the effect that she had a malignant cancer and that she should feel privileged that she had time to prepare for her death and make a will."

"In view of your behavior toward patients and colleagues there are no conditions which would enable the committee to conclude that you could safely resume practice," it said.

POLICE FIGHT RIGHT TO BARE BUTTOCKS

SYDNEY REUTERS

Australian police warned that the law would lose its bite if "mooning" became enshrined as an implied constitutional right.

A lawyer told a court in the eastern state of Queensland that his client was exercising his right to protest and was not guilty of indecency when he bared his buttocks at a police car.

But the police prosecutor said that argument was bogus and dangerous.

He told the court he could not imagine naked buttocks replacing the kangaroo and emu on Australia's Coat of Arms.

he could not imagine naked buttocks

Transvestite Sues Beauty School Over Rejection

LOS ANGELES REUTERS

A transvestite sued a Los Angeles beauty school, claiming his application was rejected when school officials realized he was not a woman.

The lawsuit, brought by a plaintiff known only as "Sandy," was the first of its kind under a 1979 city ordinance that prohibits businesses from discrimination based on sexual orientation, "Sandy"'s attorney told Reuters.

"Sandy is not required to appear as a man because she is a man or has male genitalia," said the attorney.

When he enrolled last month at the Marinello School of Beauty in Los Angeles, Sandy was perceived to be a woman, the attorney said.

After passing a test and paying a $100 fee, he was accepted to the school and told to report for classes in August. "Sandy was very happy, but her happiness did not last very long," the attorney added, referring to her client as a woman. "It had been her dream to attend beauty school."

Two hours later, after learning from Sandy's passport that she was legally a man, school officials called to say that she would not be permitted to attend classes because of concerns over which restroom he would use at school, the lawyer said.

School officials had no comment on the lawsuit.

HE'S GOING
TO HAVE A
VERY BAD DAY

TEHRAN   REUTERS

An Iranian man, convicted of rape and murder, will be executed by being thrown off a cliff in a sack, a newspaper reported.

If the unidentified man survives the fall down a rocky precipice, he will be hanged, legal experts said. He has 20 days to appeal the court sentence.

The killer was arrested last year in the northwestern city of Mashhad after "seducing" and killing his nephew, who worked as an assistant at the man's carpenter's workshop, the *Norouz* daily newspaper said.

FALL DOWN A ROCK

Measuring Nudity: You Do The Math

BADENTON | Fla.   REUTERS

A county in Florida has barred women from exposing more than 75 percent of their breasts in public, and everyone from showing more than two-thirds of their buttocks.

Now sheriff's deputies in Manatee County are wondering how they will calculate compliance.

"I don't think we'll be tape-measuring," a sheriff's spokesman told Reuters. The Manatee County Commission passed the measure in a 4-3 vote. After it takes effect on Jan. 1, violators would face $500 fines and 60 days in jail.

The spokesman said deputies would meet with state and county attorneys to determine how to interpret and enforce the law. He said they might seek a volunteer for a test arrest to see if the law holds up in court. Otherwise, deputies will focus on flagrant violators.

"It would have to be well beyond what the ordinance said. Like, naked," the spokesman said.

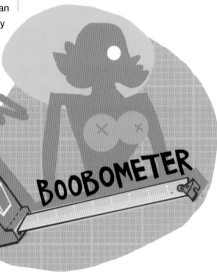

BOOBOMETER

Taxed Drug Dealer Gets Own Back

SYDNEY · REUTERS

An Australian court has given a convicted heroin dealer the all-clear to write off A$220,000 ($118,800) in stolen drug money from his tax bill.

The Federal Court ruled that as the jailed felon had earned his taxable income through selling drugs, he was likewise entitled to deduct from his taxes expenses incurred as part of his criminal endeavors.

The Perth resident was jailed for 12 years in 1996 for importing and selling heroin.

As soon as he was behind bars, Australia's meticulous tax authorities pounced and wasted no time presenting him with a A$450,000 tax bill based on what the court proceedings had revealed about the man's estimated illicit income.

The man fired back with a claim to deduct the A$220,000 he said he had buried in the garden of his daughter's home and which he intended to use to buy more drugs. He said other criminals had stolen the money when he went to make a deal.

He had already won an earlier court case but the Australian Taxation Office appealed.

CRIMINAL ENDEAVORS

SMOKING WEED ON SCHOOL TRIP NOT A CRIME?

ROME REUTERS

An Italian court has ruled that taking 40 joints of hashish on a school trip is not a crime.

The marijuana was for personal use since the 17-year-old student planned to share it with two fellow students and a teacher, the appeals court judge said.

Under Italian law, selling marijuana is a crime, but possession for personal use is not.

"It could easily have been consumed during the many days of the trip," *Corriere della Sera* daily quoted the court ruling as saying.

"Wild Party Girls" Video Brings $5 Million Judgment

SAN MARCOS | Texas   REUTERS

A Texas woman who was videotaped taking off her top at a spring break party won a $5 million judgment from the producers of "Wild Party Girls" videos after she spotted herself in a TV ad for the tapes.

The 22-year-old senior at Southwest Texas State University sued Arco Media, the Florida-based producers of the risqué videos made famous in late night TV ads.

She took action after her picture appeared in a TV advertisement for the videos broadcast on cable networks.

"She never signed a consent to have anybody film it," said her attorney. "Quite frankly, she was too drunk to legally give a valid consent."

The state district court in Hays County, Texas, entered the judgment this week after Arco failed to respond to the suit.

In previous cases, courts have ruled that there is no expectation of privacy in a public place and have upheld the right of companies to videotape the actions of women who bare their breasts, and more, at events like Mardi Gras.

WOMEN WHO BARE THEIR BREASTS

VIDEOS

iews up
omen's skirts

MAN FREE TO SELL VIDEOS SHOT UP SKIRTS

TORONTO REUTERS

A man who sells amateur videos that provide views up women's skirts has been under police surveillance for two months, but authorities said there was little they could do as there were no identifiable victims.

Police in Canada's most populous city have been investigating the man, but have not laid charges because the law does not adequately address surreptitious videotaping, a detective sergeant said.

"We've viewed the video and we're trying to determine what appropriate criminal charges can be laid," he said. "We're trying to get some new laws written to cover some of the areas that aren't covered. ... This is just the first of various (videotaping) situations that are cropping up."

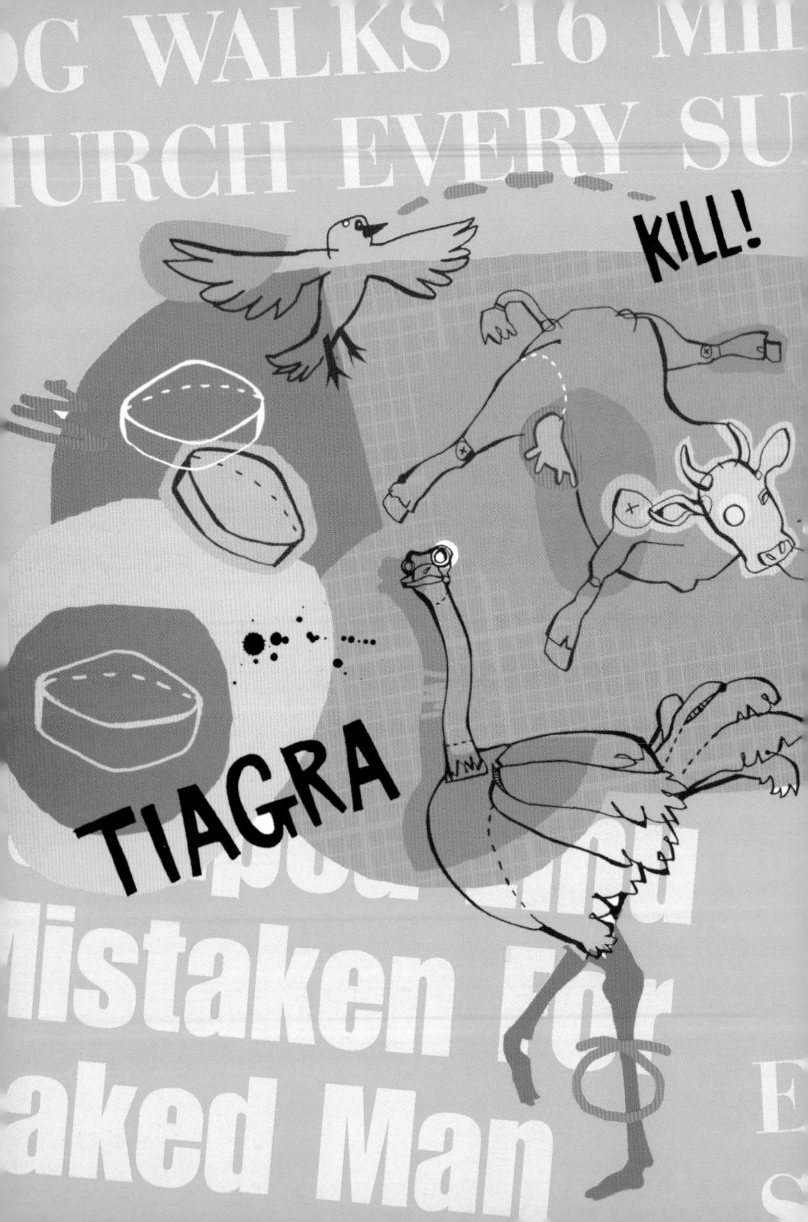

G WALKS 16
URCH EVERY
KILL!
TIAGRA
istaken
aked Man

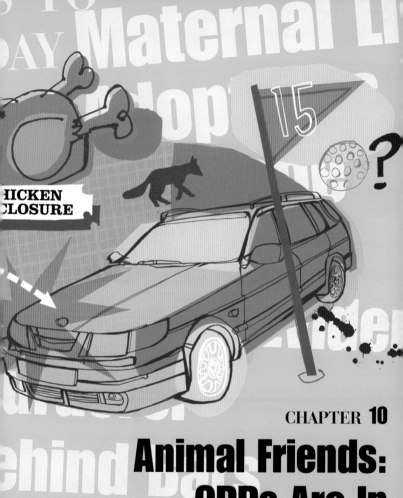

CHAPTER **10**

Animal Friends: ODDs Are In Their Favor

DOG WALKS 16 MILES TO CHURCH EVERY SUNDAY

LISBON REUTERS

Unlike many humans, Preta the dog goes to church every Sunday—and even walks 16 miles to get there.

Every Sunday for the last three years, the pooch has headed out of her owner's home in the northern Portuguese town of Sobrado at 5 a.m., *Correio da Manha* newspaper reported.

A former stray, Preta—Portuguese for "black"—walks alone to a church in neighboring Ermesinde to take her usual place next to the altar in time for 7:30 a.m. mass. Whenever worshippers stand up or sit down, Preta does the same.

Once mass is over, she usually walks back home. Sometimes Preta will return in a car—but only with a human she knows, the newspaper said.

Congregations have grown at the church as many people come just to see Preta, *Correio da Manha* said.

Well, Here's Your Problem Right Here, Ma'am

DHAKA   REUTERS

A Bangladeshi snake charmer called in to find two serpents in a suburban home near the capital unearthed over 3,000 deadly cobras and hundreds of eggs.

Police and local newspapers said the snake charmer captured more than 3,500 young cobras at two houses in Narayanganj near Dhaka.

The find, however, triggered panic among neighbors who fled their homes, police said.

Newspapers said the charmer was called in by a man whose wife had found two large cobras on their property.

Helped by his assistants, the snake charmer dug beneath the floors of two houses and unearthed the slithering stockpile.

SLITHERING
STOCKPILE

ELDERLY MAN HAS SCARE WITH ALLIGATORS

PALM HARBOR | Fla.   REUTERS

An elderly Florida man was shocked this week when he woke up in the pond behind his house staring into the faces of many alligators, police said.

The 77-year-old man said he believed he had been sleepwalking before dawn when he stumbled down an embankment and into the water.

Frail, and with a reconstructed knee, he was unable to pull himself out of the muck, so he shouted for help. A neighbor summoned help about 5 a.m.

At first police saw the crowd of alligators, but didn't see the man until he shouted, "I'm where your light is."

reconstructed

knee

CROWD OF
ALLIGATORS

Maternal Lioness Adopts Its Fifth Baby Antelope

NAIROBI REUTERS

It's nurture over nature for a lioness in Kenya who keeps choosing to dote on baby antelope rather than devour them.

Kamuniak, a lioness in northern Kenya's Samburu National Park, has adopted her fifth new-born oryx this year, a Kenya Wildlife Service warden told Reuters.

The oryx is a type of African antelope more likely to be viewed by lions as lunch than a little one to mother. Kamuniak, whose name means "the blessed one" in the local Samburu language, has been adopting oryxes since the start of the year.

On each occasion she has tried to protect the calves from other predators and even allowed their natural mothers to come feed them. But eventually the calves escape with the help of their natural mothers, are rescued by park wardens or in one case made into a snack by a male lion while Kamuniak napped.

The wardens think Kamuniak's adoption of the little calf nicknamed Naisimari ("taken by force") took place at the weekend after they saw the two together.

"She must have adopted her yesterday because they are in harmony," the Samburu warden said.

Naisimari's natural mother has been seen following her offspring and its unlikely surrogate parent at a distance.

Zookeepers Suspended For Eating Animals

BERLIN REUTERS

Two zookeepers in a small northwest German town have been suspended and put under police investigation for eating the zoo's animals, police said.

A police spokesman in Recklinghausen, north of Cologne, said the keepers in a section of the zoo popular with small children had slaughtered and barbecued five Tibetan mountain chickens and two Cameroonian sheep.

"The animals were in the 'pet' zoo where all the children would go to stroke them," the spokesman said. Suspicious zoo managers called police after the animals disappeared.

PET CHICKEN FALLS FOUL OF LAW

AMSTERDAM REUTERS

An Italian tourist cried foul after being arrested for taking his pet chicken for a walk in the Netherlands, which is grappling with a bird flu outbreak.

The man, who was touring Europe with his chicken, was taken to a police station where a vet culled his pet. The man was not fined but he had to pay for the vet and an animal ambulance.

"The man said he didn't know anything about the avian flu and a transport ban in the Netherlands. He left disappointed and said he would complain at the Italian consulate," a spokesman for police in the western town of IJmuiden told Reuters.

FISH-SNIFFING CAT HELPS BATTLE SMUGGLERS

MOSCOW   REUTERS

Move over bomb-sniffing dogs, here comes Rusik, the fish-sniffing cat!

Russian police battling fish smugglers have deployed a cat to sniff out contraband, including Caspian Sea sturgeon which produce Russia's world famous caviar.

A police control post in the southern Stavropol region adopted Rusik one year ago and it now helps officers conduct spot checks on vehicles, the Itar-Tass news agency reported. The cat had distinguished itself with an outstanding nose for fish.

"The cat finds it in any hiding place," Itar-Tass quoted a police spokesman in Stavropol as saying, adding that Rusik was fed on confiscated fish.

CONFISCATED FISH

Escaped Emu Mistaken For Naked Man

HAMBURG | Germany   REUTERS

An escaped emu caused confusion in Hamburg after a woman called police to report what she thought was a bare-chested man with two big white dots on his forehead staring into her window, police said.

The large, flightless Australian bird resembling an ostrich has been on the run from a local zoo.

"The woman heard someone tapping at the window at night and when she looked out she saw a head with two big eyes and a bare chest," a Hamburg police spokesman said.

Officers said they knew there was an emu on the run and put two and two together after they found no one suspicious.

"We're still looking for either a naked man with huge eyes or an emu," the spokesman added.

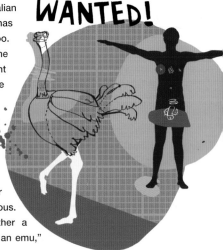

WANTED!

Utility Says Keep Your Chickens Grounded

SAN FRANCISCO   REUTERS

Pacific Gas & Electric asked the public not to launch any more chickens into its power lines.

The utility is eager to avoid a repeat of last weekend's escapade in which some San Francisco prankster tied about 100 helium balloons to a chicken and sent it aloft where it became tangled in local power lines.

The chicken, though uninjured, was left dangling for about three hours while PG&E crews brought it back to earth. The rescue effort required cutting power to about 5,000 people.

A PG&E spokesman said, "It's pretty outrageous somebody would do this and that's why we're asking the public today not to do something like this in the future."

The chicken is being put up for adoption by a local animal shelter, which has also launched an investigation to find those responsible.

FOX STEALS BALLS

STOCKHOLM REUTERS

A fox snapped up two balls hit from the seventh tee on to the fairway by players in a tournament at Gronhogen golf course on the island of Oland off Sweden's southeastern coast, TT news agency said.

The players saw the fox run off into nearby woods and when the tournament director consulted the rule book he found no guidance about how to proceed.

He chose to allow the players to drop new balls near where they had stopped. The fox, hoarding food for the winter, had apparently mistaken the golf balls for bird eggs.

Ferret Causes Mayhem On Train

LONDON REUTERS

A hungry ferret caused chaos on a commuter train in central England, jumping aboard at a station and leaping from passenger to passenger before ducking into the engineer's cab and devouring his lunch.

"It ran up and down the train causing more than a little consternation—although it is hard to say if the ferret or the passengers were more frightened," a company spokeswoman said.

"It then got into the driver's cab and ate his lunch—a cheese sandwich I think—before he realized what was going on," she told Reuters.

The quick-thinking engineer radioed ahead for experts from the Royal Society for the Prevention of Cruelty to Animals to meet the train, capture the ferret and remove it so the journey could continue.

Hero Bird's Evidence Lands Murderer Behind Bars

A hero cockatoo slain trying to protect its master from knife-wielding assailants proved the star witness in the trial of one of its owner's killers.

Daniel Torres was found guilty of murdering Kevin Butler. Prosecutors have said DNA evidence extracted from the bird's beak as well as blood trails caused when the bird violently pecked the assailants were key pieces of evidence that led to the conviction.

According to evidence presented in court, Torres and another suspect broke into Butler's home. During a struggle in Butler's living room, the white-crested cockatoo, named Bird after the basketball great Larry Bird, swooped down on the attackers, clawed at their skin and pecked at their heads, said prosecutor George West.

West said blood found in Bird's beak and at the scene of the crime linked Torres to the murder.

Bird may have wounded Torres, but the protective parrot paid the price for trying to take on two armed foes. Bird had its leg cut off and was found dead in the kitchen of Butler's home—apparently stabbed to death by a fork in the back.

It took a Dallas jury less than an hour to find Torres guilty. He was sentenced to life in prison.

New Berlin Wall To Be Erected—For Frogs

BERLIN REUTERS

Cash-strapped Berlin is spending about $475,000 to build a network of walls and tunnels to protect frogs crossing a busy road.

The plan has angered Berlin taxpayers because it coincides with the closures of swimming pools, kindergartens and other public services as the German capital cuts costs.

Despite its debt of almost $50 million at the end of 2002, Berlin is building 15 tunnels to give frogs safe passage on their way to a nearby lake, wildlife protection officials said.

Construction is under way in Pankow, eastern Berlin, and includes a 650-yard concrete wall to guide frogs toward the tunnels.

"I'm all for protecting animals, but this really is a utopian scheme," said the head of Berlin's taxpayer association. "It's a colossal waste of money."

TURNING TO VIAGRA TO INCREASE TIGER BIRTHS

BEIJING   REUTERS

Chinese zoos will give Viagra to South China tigers with no sex drive in a last-ditch effort to raise the numbers of the highly endangered species.

A pair of male tigers showing "no sexual desire" at a zoo in China's southern province of Sichuan will be the first to receive doses of the anti-impotence drug, the Xinhua news agency said.

Cage life was responsible for their infertility, it said.

Ten zoos around the country are home to 49 South China tigers, a rare species experts say could become extinct because they are raised in isolation, live in unsuitable artificial surroundings and because of inbreeding, Xinhua said.

The annual meeting of the South China Tiger Protection Society found that six years of protection work had done little to help reduce the danger of extinction of the big cats, it said.

There are only 20-30 wild South China tigers remaining, Xinhua said.

Scientists have also considered using Viagra to boost the sex drive of captive Giant Pandas, another endangered species that has trouble mating.

One Chinese research institute even tried to educate impotent pandas about sex by showing them videos of other pandas mating.

Car Smashed By Falling Cow

VIENNA　REUTERS

A cow toppled off its lofty Alpine pasture and crashed onto the hood of an Austrian couple's car in the picturesque province of Salzburg, police said.

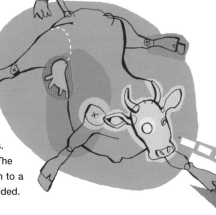

The cow did not survive the fall off the so-called gallery—an open-sided roof over roads to protect people from avalanches.

The car was a write-off. The driver's wife was hurt and taken to a hospital, the Salzburg police added.

THE CAR WAS A WRITE-OFF

SWAN LAKE FROM HELL

OSLO   REUTERS

A Norwegian swan named Oscar, famous for his short temper, attacked an elderly woman, biting her bottom, dragging her into a lake and ducking her twice before letting go.

"Oscar came flying from across the other side of the lake and bit me in the buttocks before dragging me about five yards into the water and under," the woman told Reuters.

"He only let me go when my daughter started to throw rocks."

She said the attack happened as she, her daughter and three small grandchildren were strolling in a nature reserve near the southwestern city of Kristiansand.

Police and medical staff were quickly on the scene and Oscar was immediately put down by police.

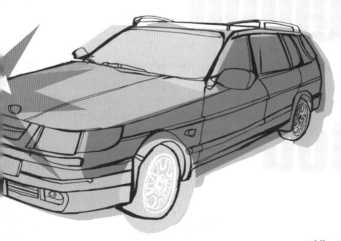

NUDE PROTEST

PAMPLONA | Spain REUTERS

Animal rights activists stripped naked to protest the running of bulls through the streets of Pamplona, denouncing one of Spain's most famous traditions as cruel to animals.

Activists from all over Western Europe had planned to run nude along the route for the annual bull runs, but police in the northern Spanish city said the protest was unauthorized and blocked their way.

About 20 men and women went ahead with the protest near the city center however, stripping completely. Some put on plastic horns or fake bull's heads. They were joined by scores of other protesters who kept on all or part of their clothing.

Woman Shares Car With Rat

OSLO REUTERS

A terrified Norwegian woman shared her car with a rat for two weeks after failing to lure the animal into a trap.

The six-inch-long rat, which sneaked out of a garbage bag and built a nest under the dashboard with discarded Norwegian crown bills and old receipts, was not tempted by a mousetrap loaded with cheese, sausage or minced beef.

"I'm disgusted. Imagine, I drove with that big, ugly thing right underneath my legs," the 35-year-old consultant from southeast Norway told Reuters.

The rat was finally killed when the woman laced the trap with liver pate.

"I'm laughing now that the beast is dead, but I was really scared," she said.

King Calls For End To Live Animal Targets

PHNOM PENH | Cambodia   REUTERS

Cambodia's King Norodom Sihanouk has called for a halt of the use of live animal targets at the country's only shooting range outside Phnom Penh.

Cambodia's international image was being tarnished by the shooting range's policy of allowing tourists and other visitors to shoot live cows, buffalo, goats and chickens, Sihanouk said in a letter to the Interior Ministry.

"In foreign countries, they take wooden or plastic targets for shooting. In Cambodia, they take live animals such as chickens and cows to be shot dead," said the letter, published in a monthly bulletin released by the palace.

"Please check and curb such things in order not to defame our nation in the international arena," the king said.

A staff member at the government-run shooting range, where everything from automatic weapons to rocket-propelled grenades is available, told Reuters that visitors had not been allowed to shoot live animal targets for almost a year.

He said the practice was once quite popular, especially among wealthy Japanese tourists who would pay $5 for a chicken and $100-300 for a cow or water buffalo, depending on the size.

"I once saw a goat used as a target for a B40 rocket. There was nothing left afterwards," he said.

MONKEY VISITS PIZZERIA

BERLIN   REUTERS

An escaped circus monkey dropped into a pizzeria in a small German town and vandalized the ladies toilet even though the owner had tried to pacify the animal with salad and rolls.

The owner was standing in front of the counter of his pizzeria in the northern town of Lehre when "Lala," a one-and-a-half-foot-tall Rhesus monkey, entered through the front door.

The owner and a cook used lettuce to lure Lala into the women's toilet, where they fed the monkey rolls to keep it calm.

But Lala tossed all the paper towels into the sink and turned on the tap, flooding both toilets, the kitchen and part of the dining room.

Man Entraps Neighbor's Dog With Taped Barks

BERLIN   REUTERS

A German used recorded barking to provoke a neighbor's dog to respond so he could report the animal for disturbing the peace, police said.

"The man evidently didn't like the dog and wanted to make it bark more so he could report it," a police spokesman in the northern town of Harrislee said.

After the man complained to police about the German shepherd, the neighbor discovered a speaker hidden in his hedge attached to a cable leading to the man's house. He alerted police, who found the system was rigged up to play dog barks and sounds of tongue clicks meant to attract canines.

Cop Breathes Life Into Stricken Dog

WEST BRIDGEWATER | Mass.　　REUTERS

A police officer brought a stricken dog back to life by performing mouth-to-mouth resuscitation on her furry muzzle after she was hit by a car, the officer said.

The patrolman said Cinnamon the pit bull terrier was technically dead and her owner was "hysterical" when he arrived at the scene of the accident.

"She had been hit in the chest area. All four of her legs went out and her heart was not beating. She was dead," the officer told Reuters.

The officer, who owns a dog himself, immediately started to perform cardiopulmonary resuscitation (CPR) on the lifeless pooch, alternately pressing on her chest and breathing into her muzzle.

"It took me seven or eight tries but to my amazement, she opened her eyes and started breathing," he said, adding that he then transported Cinnamon to a local animal hospital.

"She's fine. She has some nerve damage but no broken bones. It's a miracle," he said.

"IT'S A MIRACLE"

VICIOUS CROW KILLED AFTER TERRORIZING CITY

FRANKFURT REUTERS

A vicious crow which terrorized a Frankfurt suburb and provoked a fight between two residents has been shot and killed, the city's environmental authority said.

"We're usually here to protect birds but this was different. The crow had been making targeted attacks on people, we don't know why," said the head of Frankfurt's nature conservation authority, which ordered the shooting.

In a reminder of director Alfred Hitchcock's classic horror film "The Birds," the crow had been attacking people for five weeks, swooping down and pecking at their heads.

The bird also caused at least one fight. A man trying to protect himself by throwing a plastic bag at the crow was beaten up by a passing motorist who thought the bag had been aimed at his car.

The Stuff Of Urban Legends

AMSTERDAM   REUTERS

A pet python missing for two months made its reappearance by scaring a Dutch woman when it slithered out of her toilet bowl.

The constrictor snake, which kills its prey by coiling around it and squeezing, had been on the loose after breaking out of its terrarium in a town near the port city of Rotterdam, Dutch news agency ANP said.

As police and vets came to catch the six-foot-long fugitive python, it slid under a bathtub that they had to demolish.

The snake was returned to its owner, but local residents were unhappy to hear the owner admit that a second pet python, this one almost three feet long, had also escaped and was still on the loose.

Would-Be Rescuer Feared Killed By Whale Tail Blow

WELLINGTON   REUTERS

A New Zealand man trying to free a 50-foot humpback whale ensnared in lobster pot ropes is missing and presumed dead after being hit by the whale's tail, police said.

The 38-year-old man had gone to the aid of a whale in waters near the popular whale-watching town of Kaikoura, 90 miles south of Wellington.

"He was trying to cut the rope free from the whale's tail and the whale lifted its tail and struck him," a Kaikoura police sergeant told Reuters.

Young Dog Swims 10 Miles After Going Overboard

LONDON   REUTERS

A young black Labrador paddled for 10 miles dodging ferries, oil tankers and yachts to reach land after falling overboard from his master's boat off the southern English coast.

Two-year-old Todd's six-hour marathon surprised canine experts and delighted his owner, newspapers said.

The owner, who spent four hours searching for Todd after discovering his canine crewmember had jumped ship, said it was a miracle he had survived.

"He swam across the waves, across the currents to get home," he said. "I am so pleased to see him, he is like a child to me."

Pet and master were finally reunited after Todd swam up the River Beaulieu in Hampshire. The dog clambered asore, and police scanned a microchip in the dog's ear.

"HEALTH FREAK" POLAR BEAR STEALS TOOTHPASTE

OSLO REUTERS

A polar bear and apparent health freak has stolen toothpaste and vitamin pills after breaking into a tourist camp in the Norwegian Arctic, but bizarrely left food untouched.

"Maybe he felt he had bad breath after eating seal all summer," joked the owner of Svalbard Wildlife Service, the tour operator whose camp was trampled.

Fourteen tourists and guides from Norway, Sweden and Italy came to the camp on the Arctic island of Spitsbergen last week to find the bear had knocked over tents, bitten through a tube of toothpaste and sucked out its contents.

Polar bears' teeth are often yellow, unlike their snow-white fur. The bear, probably aged two, had also popped vitamin-C pills. Dried meat hanging from the roof of one large tent and other food within reach were untouched.

popped vitamin-C pills

Crocodile Luggage Left On Bus

SYDNEY REUTERS

Australia's quirky Northern Territory has more crocodiles than humans, but they don't normally take the bus.

The driver told the Australian Associated Press news agency he did not notice his reptilian passenger until a woman passenger pointed under his seat.

"I've got no idea where he came from," the driver said near Darwin, capital of the northern Australian region that covers an area five times the size of Britain stretching from tropical rainforest to desert.

"I believe someone must have taken him into the bus thinking that they'd take him somewhere and maybe he was too strong for them to hold so he disappeared under the seat and they've done a quiet exit and left me with the crocodile," he said. "It's just one of those things that happen in the Territory."

The 30-inch crocodile had its jaws taped shut but still managed to scratch a police officer's hand when it was taken into custody before being handed to game wardens.

30-inch crocodile

DOG GIVES FLASHER HIS COME-UPPANCE

ZAGREB REUTERS

A drunken Croat flasher got more excitement than he bargained for when he pushed his penis through a woman's fence and her dog bit it, local newspapers said.

The visibly drunk man was walking down the street and started swearing and shouting at the woman for no reason. He then shoved his penis through her fence, unaware her dog was on the other side, police said.

The bitten man complained to police about the incident, but received no sympathy.

The 36-year-old was taken to a nearby hospital with light injuries but was later sent home. He will be charged with "insulting the moral feelings of citizens" and "violation of public order."

Man Fails Test, Dog Passes

BERLIN REUTERS

A German man lost his driving license after failing an alcohol test but his dog passed with flying colors, police in the western city of Koblenz said.

Police said the 47-year-old man failed to perform any of the required actions, only to be upstaged by his West Highland white terrier who followed all of the commands, including a 360-degree turn as his master staggered and fell.

At the conclusion of the uneven contest, the superviser announced, "Man: fail; dog: pass."

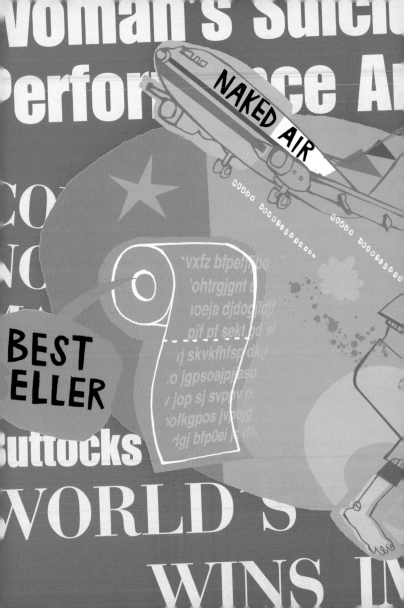

ART?

COUNTY SAYS NO TO NAKED MACBETH

SANFORD | Fla.   REUTERS

Seminole County commissioners in Florida did not mind that a local nightclub was serving up eye of newt, toe of frog, wool of bat and tongue of dog.

What they did object to was the fact that the three witches in the club's version of Shakespeare's "Macbeth" were played by naked dancers.

The commissioners unanimously passed a law banning nudity in places that sell alcohol, closing a loophole in the public decency ordinance which the Club Juana nightclub in Casselberry had exploited to stage the naked witch scene.

The ordinance had required strippers to cover at least part of their breasts and buttocks but exempted theatrical performances.

The club has already staged several performances of a revue, "Les Femmes Fatales," featuring the witch scene, a sword dance and excerpts from the Marquis de Sade's "Philosophy in the Bedroom."

Woman's Suicide Taken For Performance Art

BERLIN   REUTERS

Visitors to an offbeat Berlin arts center thought a dead woman on the ground was a performance art act rather than a suicide, police said.

Authorities said the 24-year-old woman, who apparently leapt from a window, discussed suicide in a videotaped interview with a group of artists the day before.

"A group of visitors to the center at first thought the body lying on the ground at the art center was part of an art performance," said a police spokeswoman. "It took a while before anyone realized it was not an act but a suicide."

Artists at the Tacheles art center had videotaped the woman the evening before when she told of her suicide plans. They tried to talk her out of it and drove her home, but she returned to the arts workshop later in the evening.

discussed
suicide
in a videotaped
interview

WORLD'S WORST POET WINS IMMORTALITY

LONDON   REUTERS

A Scottish poet so bad he was often asked to perform just so the audience could laugh at him will have his verse etched in stone in the city where he worked.

William Topaz McGonagall, who died in 1902, has gained posthumous recognition in the Scottish city of Dundee, which plans to mark the centenary of his death by engraving part of one his poems on a walkway by the river Tay.

"His poetry is so bad it's memorable," said Niall Scott, director of City of Discovery Campaign, the organization behind the plan.

"Dundee has recognized the need to honor McGonagall as somebody absolutely dedicated to the art of awful poetry."

"No one can surpass him for being the worst poet," said Mervyn Rolfe, chairman of City of Discovery Campaign and a member of the Dundee-based McGonagall Appreciation Society. "He doesn't care how many words there are in the line as long as the last words rhyme, so the meter is appalling."

That was also the opinion of many of McGonagall's contemporaries, who responded to his efforts by inventing "poet-baiting"—a form of public entertainment in which the poet performed while the audience jeered.

Affection for the self-styled tragedian of the Victorian age has grown since his demise, culminating in the plan to engrave the first two verses of "The Railway Bridge of the Silvery Tay" in the ground near the bridge as long overdue recognition.

A fine example of McGonagall's art, the poem begins:

"Beautiful Railway Bridge of the Silvery Tay!
With your numerous arches and pillars in so grand array
And your central girders, which seem to the eye
To be almost towering to the sky..."

Radio "War Correspondent" Has Cover Blown

MBABANE   REUTERS

Listeners to Swaziland's state-run radio station thought it had its own correspondent in Baghdad covering the war—until legislators spotted him in parliament at the weekend.

"Why are they lying to the nation that the man is in Iraq, when he is here in Swaziland broadcasting out of a broom closet?" a member of parliament demanded of the information minister in the House of Assembly.

The minister said he would investigate the matter.

The correspondent presented "live reports" purportedly from Baghdad. The program host frequently expressed concerns about his well-being and once advised him to "find a cave somewhere to be safe from missiles."

The station declined comment.

Burning Yule Log Wins Christmas TV Ratings

LOS ANGELES REUTERS

Show them nothing, and they will watch.

A television program showing only a Yule log burning in a fireplace–accompanied by a soundtrack of seasonal songs– was the highest rated morning show in New York City on Christmas Day, the Nielsen television ratings service said.

Titled simply "Yule Log," the show attracted about 611,000 viewers to WPIX Channel 11 to finish No. 1 for the time period from 8 a.m. to 10 a.m., Nielsen said. The closest competitor was WABC Channel 7's "Good Morning America," which attracted about 532,000 viewers.

The general manager of WPIX, which is owned by the Tribune Co., said the two-hour Yule log program was a remastered version of a WPIX staple from 1966 to 1989.

"Every year we get so many requests from people to bring back the Yule log," she said. "People are looking for tradition. They're clinging to tradition this year. We thought this would be the ultimate in comfort television ... The fire kept you extra warm this year."

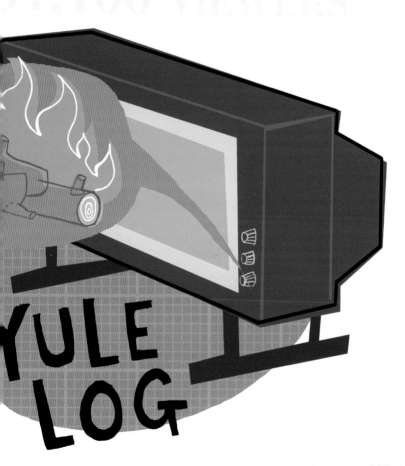

YULE
LOG

BING CROSBY HIT KEEPS TEENS ON THE MOVE

SYDNEY REUTERS

An Australian shopping center has found a novel way to deter teenage loiterers—playing loud Bing Crosby music.

The late American crooner has hit a sour note with youths with his 1938 hit My Heart is Taking Lessons, which is being played repeatedly at the entrance to the Warrawong shopping center in southern New South Wales.

Sydney's *Daily Telegraph* newspaper reported that the center was also using pink fluorescent lights that highlight pimples.

"All the people from Warrawong High used to hang here after school - now you don't see them," a 14-year-old youth told the newspaper.

pink fluorescent lights

Hens Saved From Execution On Stage

BERLIN REUTERS

Two hens escaped public execution during performance of a play when animal lovers stormed the stage, a spokeswoman for an animal shelter in the south German town of Wuerzburg said.

The fowl were due to be killed as part of a performance of "The Slaughter of Two Chickens" by German playwright Alf Poss, but animal welfare activists struck before any feathers flew.

"It was our duty to rescue the hens and ensure their welfare," a spokeswoman for the animal shelter said.

The theater director defended his production, saying it was meant as a comment on Third World hunger.

"In the end, it's all about the tension," he said. The play required the slaughter of two chickens per performance—a total of 48 for the play's season.

Killing chickens without a license carries a penalty of up to three years imprisonment or a fine for cruelty to animals.

Restorers Take Corsets Off Bernini Beauties

ROME REUTERS

Restoration works in a Roman church have revealed two bare-breasted beauties designed by Bernini but hidden behind bronze "corsets" for more than 100 years, officials said.

The figures, representing truth and charity, were designed by Gian Lorenzo Bernini and sculpted with his assistants in the 1660s for the Baroque church of Sant'Isidoro, but later censored by religious leaders.

"The nudes were a bit too provocative for the Victorians, so they were covered with bronze corsets in 1863," the church's director of restoration works told Reuters.

"We decided to bare all," she said.

The striptease revealed two white marble figures squeezing their breasts seductively.

Blind Psychic Gropes Buttocks To See Future

BERLIN   REUTERS

Forget palm reading. A blind German psychic claimed he could read people's futures by feeling their naked buttocks.

Clairvoyant Ulf Buck, 39, claims that people's backsides have lines like those on the palm of the hand which can be read to reveal much about their character and destiny.

"The bottom is much more intense —it has a much stronger power of expression than the hand in my experience," Buck told Reuters. "It goes on developing throughout your life."

By running his fingers along a number of lines on the surface of a client's posterior, he says he can tell them about their future monetary success, family life, health and happiness.

He says lines representing success, career and artistic ability extend inwards from the outer extremities of the buttocks, while a further five lines radiate outwards.

"I began on a circle of friends and the circle grew," Buck said. "I am not a new-age freak. I treat people with great care and conscientiousness."

Buck, who lives in the northern village of Meldorf, northwest of Hamburg, says all types come to him to have their bottoms read.

He sees his blindness as a great asset, not least because it means customers do not risk having their identities revealed.

He is quick to shoot down any suggestion that his buttock groping might be motivated by anything other than a genuine desire to probe people's futures.

"I do not need to feel bottoms for my own pleasure. My wife is quite beautiful enough for me," he said.

Taking Off, And Taking it Off

HOUSTON   REUTERS

On Naked-Air, seatbelts aren't the only things coming off once the pilot switches off the sign.

Passengers aboard a May 3 chartered flight from Miami to Cancun, Mexico, dubbed "Naked-Air," will be free to drop their pants, shed their bras and underwear and move about the cabin au naturel.

Castaways Travel, a Houston-area travel agency that specializes in "clothing-optional trips," is offering what it proudly bills as the world's first ever all-nude flight for $499 round-trip.

"Once the aircraft reaches cruising altitude, you will be free to enjoy the flight clothes-free," the agency's Web site says.

But those thinking about engaging in monkey business on the trip are warned: "Inappropriate behavior is not condoned for this nude flight."

Seats aboard the chartered Boeing 727-200 jet are reserved for the first 170 passengers, and the destination is an all-inclusive "Nude Week" vacation at the El Dorado Resort & Spa in Cancun.

FIRST ALL-NUDE
FLIGHT FOR $499

BERMUDA TOURISM ADS SHOT IN OTHER EDENS

HAMILTON REUTERS

Bermuda, the picturesque Atlantic island famed for its pink beaches, has admitted using pictures shot in other locales in tourism ads, a newspaper reported.

Three photographs in the advertising campaign were stock images that were not shot in the British colony, the island's *Royal Gazette* newspaper quoted a Department of Tourism official as saying.

One features a model shot on a beach in Hawaii. Another shows a scuba diver surrounded by fish thought to have been taken in the Seychelles. The third shows a woman swimming with a dolphin photographed in Florida, the newspaper reported.

"The images in question, you could never tell where in the world they are, and they portray more of a feeling and position for Bermuda in our profile of sophisticated contemporaries. Stock images are used all the time in the industry," the travel official told the newspaper.

DRIVERS ROCK 'N' ROLL WITH KARAOKE CAR

SHANGHAI   REUTERS

China's gridlocked drivers will be able to sing their blues away next year after the country's only privately owned car maker rolls out a car equipped with karaoke gear.

China Geely Group said its new model, the Geely Beauty Leopard, would retail for 150,000 yuan ($18,000) and come with a phone, karaoke machine and other bells and whistles, such as navigation gear based on the global positioning system.

Now, THAT'S Reality!

DUBLIN   REUTERS

An Irish reality television show nearly sank without trace after the ship carrying contestants around the country's treacherous coastline hit the rocks and broke up.

Terrified contestants taking part in state broadcaster RTE's "Cabin Fever" program were winched to safety by helicopter after the boat that was supposed to be their home for eight weeks ran aground near Tory Island, Donegal, in northwest Ireland.

A producer with the company making the program—flagged as the Irish television event of the summer—said all precautions had been taken, the ship having been thoroughly checked before setting out and the crew trained in sea survival.

"I have no idea how it happened," he told RTE.

He said the incident had not been caught on film as the camera crew had not been on duty.

AUGHT ON FILM

"Cabin Fever"

TOILET PAPER NOVELS HIT STALLS

FRANKFURT REUTERS

Germans who like to read on the toilet no longer need to take newspapers in with them, but can instead turn to novels and poems printed on toilet paper, a German publisher said.

"We want our books to be used. That's our philosophy," said Georges Hemmerstoffer, of the Klo-Verlag which publishes the toilet paper literature. About half of all people like to read on the toilet, he said.

Poems by German literary giants Heinrich Heine and Christian Morgenstern, as well as tales and detective stories, could be found on the toilet rolls, Hemmerstoffer told Reuters at the Frankfurt book fair.

Each text was printed several times on one roll, so that readers could enjoy the stories, but actually use the paper and still leave behind some entertaining reading for the next toilet visitor.

printed on
toilet paper

Paper Falls For Gag In Tabloid

BEIJING   REUTERS

Beijing's most popular newspaper has unwittingly republished a bogus story about the U.S. Congress threatening to skip town for Memphis or Charlotte unless Washington builds them a new Capitol building with a retractable dome.

The source? America's celebrated spoof tabloid, the *Onion*.

The Beijing *Evening News*, which claims a circulation of 1.25 million, translated portions of the *Onion*'s tall tale word-for-word on its international news page.

The reprinted version of the article, which parodies Congress as a Major League Baseball squad, also copied the *Onion*'s would-be blueprint for a new legislative home that resembles a ballpark.

"Don't get us wrong: We love the drafty old building," the *Onion* jestingly quoted House Speaker Dennis Hastert as saying.

"But the hard reality is, it's no longer suitable for a world-class legislative branch. The sight lines are bad, there aren't enough concession stands or bathrooms, and the parking is miserable."

The spoof from the brazen entertainment tabloid apparently took in the *Evening News*.

"The story was written by one of our freelance writers," an editor at the *Evening News* told Reuters. "His stuff has been pretty much reliable before."

The editor said he had received other calls from readers about the article. "They were also suspicious of the contents."

Told the story came from the *Onion* and was not true, the editor said, "We would first have to check that out. If it's indeed fake, I'm sure there will be some form of correction."

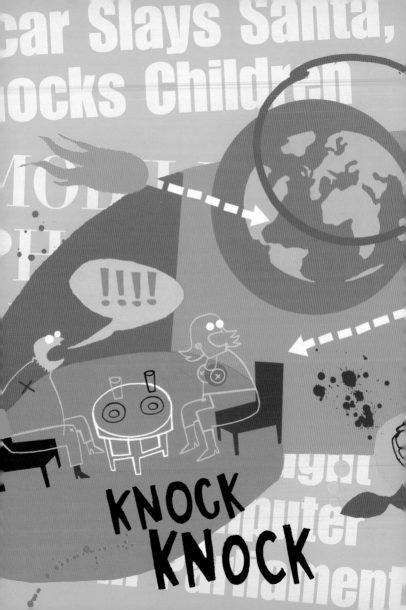

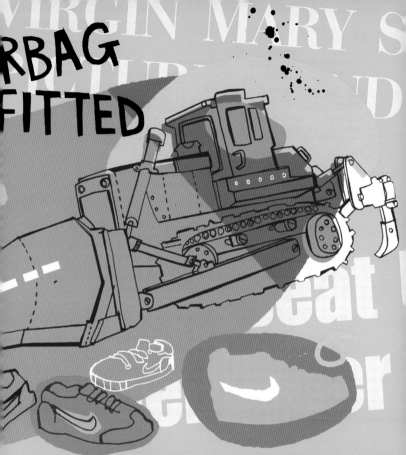

CHAPTER **12**
Potpourri: Too ODD To Categorize

Man Complains Bad Rope Spoiled His Suicide

BUCHAREST   REUTERS

A Romanian man plans to complain to consumer authorities about the poor quality of a rope he used in a failed attempt to hang himself, Romanian papers reported.

"You can't even die in this country," the 45-year-old man was quoted as saying in the daily *Adevarul*.

The newspaper said the man's relatives found him hanging from a tree in his garden and managed to cut the rope with a knife. The man said he would file a complaint with the Consumer Protection Authority about the quality of the rope, which was easily cut, as soon as he was released from the hospital.

Vicar Slays Santa, Shocks Children

LONDON   REUTERS

A British vicar reduced young children to tears and stunned their parents when he said Santa Claus and his reindeer would burn to a crisp while delivering presents at supersonic speed.

The vicar shattered the illusions of dozens of kids when he joked in his carol service sermon that Santa and his reindeer would burn up doing 3,000 times the speed of sound as they delivered gifts to 91.8 million homes.

"I am mortified and appreciate that I have put some parents in a difficult position," he told the *Daily Telegraph*. "I love Christmas."

"AIRBAG DESK" FOR TIRED OFFICE WORKERS

BERLIN   REUTERS

A German engineer has designed a desk that converts into a giant pillow at the push of a button for flagging office workers in need of a quick snooze.

"At work I was often tempted to just lie down and take a quick afternoon nap," said the man whose "airbag table" will soon be on display at a Hamburg art gallery.

"The airbag table is designed for everyone who works hard at their desk and needs to take a quick nap," he told Reuters.

A prototype of the desk, made out of walnut, looks perfectly ordinary until a small button is pressed underneath. This activates a fan that inflates a bright orange airbag, which unfolds through an opened panel on the desktop.

But the 32-year-old designer said he hoped his invention wouldn't encourage people to work even longer hours.

"The aim isn't to keep people chained to their desks 24 hours a day," he said. "I think people should get away from their desks at some point and get a life."

inflates a bright orange airbag

Lawmaker Caught Playing Computer Game In Parliament

OSLO REUTERS

A Norwegian member of parliament apologized for playing a war game on his pocket computer while legislators around him debated the possibility of a real war in Iraq.

The lawmaker, a member of the ruling Conservative Party, was caught on a national television camera playing the game during the debate about whether Norway would take part in any U.S.-led military action against Iraq.

He said he was sorry he had been tempted to try out the new game as he was checking his handheld PC diary for the day's meetings.

"I realize it was very stupid of me. I will not do it again," he told Reuters.

real war in Iraq

MINOR TOURISM MIRACLE

"Oh you're probably
seeing your own
shadow."

VIRGIN MARY SEEN ON PICTURE WINDOW

WINNIPEG | Manitoba REUTERS

Sightings of images of the Virgin Mary on windows and walls in northern reaches of the Canadian province of Saskatchewan have produced a minor tourism miracle for the remote villages involved.

Since September, mysterious images of Mary, mother of Christ, have been reported in four villages—three of which are accessible only by airplane—spurring hundreds of people to visit.

The latest images appeared on two homes in Beauval, Saskatchewan, which has fewer than 1,000 residents. The images appear to glow at night and have been captured on video, said a woman who owns one of the homes.

She said she didn't want to tell others about the image on her picture window at first. "I told my mom ... and she said, 'Oh you're probably seeing your own shadow,' so I thought people wouldn't believe me," the woman told Reuters.

Since then more than 300 people have come from hundreds of miles around to view her window.

Bulldozer Rams Wrong Home

HOLLYWOOD | Fla.   REUTERS

A Florida couple's dinner was interrupted when a bulldozer tore down part of the roof of their house as they sat inside.

The bulldozer was set to demolish several homes in Hollywood, Florida, but it rammed into the wrong house, police said.

The couple was having dinner when the bulldozer came in through the back of their house, a police spokesman said. It hit the rental home a second time before screaming neighbors and the couple prompted the driver to stop.

"I started yelling at him, 'What the hell are you guys doing?'" the resident told the *Sun-Sentinel*.

Nearby homes in the neighborhood, 20 miles north of Miami, were scheduled to be demolished as part of a renewal project but the couple's rental home was not on the list.

"What can you say? They screwed up. They hit the wrong house," the spokesman said.

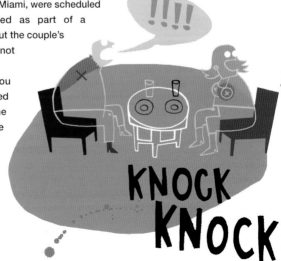

KNOCK
KNOCK

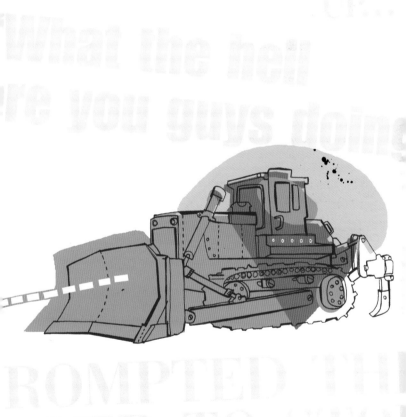

MAN STRIKES OIL, ISN'T HAPPY

BERLIN   REUTERS

A German oil delivery man who got his addresses mixed up accidentally pumped 3,000 liters of heating oil straight into a house's basement, police in the western town of Marburg said.

The mishap happened when the man attached the pump to a disused pipe at the front of the house next to the one he was supposed to deliver to.

He then pumped enough heating oil to fill around 30 bathtubs down the sawed-off pipe, completely flooding the owners' basement and ruining their belongings before spotting his mistake and alerting police.

"The house's front door is very close to that of the neighbor's, and the filler neck flap was just to the side of the door -- unfortunately it was defunct and belonged to the wrong house," said a Marburg police spokesman.

Fire services succeeded in pumping out 2,000 liters of the oily mess but a substantial amount got into the sewers and water authorities had to be called in to prevent environmental damage, police said.

"The man said he'd been delivering oil for 15 years, but he didn't think he'd been there before," the spokesman said.

Police Beat Up Undercover Colleagues At Demo

BERLIN   REUTERS

German police mistakenly beat up their own undercover detectives when a demonstration turned violent in the northern city of Hamburg.

Police were monitoring a rally of some 3,000 people protesting the demolition of illegal squatters' homes when violence broke out.

Several hundred helmet-clad riot police then clashed with the protesters, including plainclothes officers who had been shoved into the center of the crowd.

Local political leaders from the Hamburg Social Democrats investigating the matter said the officers tried to identify themselves with a password.

But communication efforts failed and riot police beat their colleagues with batons, leaving two with head injuries.

MOBILE PHONE GUNS SEIZED

ROUEN | France   REUTERS

French police said they had seized two lethal mobile phones capable of shooting four bullets, with the digital touchpads used as triggers.

The black telephones, identical to normal mobile phones on the outside, were discovered in a raid on a suspected gangster's home in the northern town of Rouen.

The fake phones came apart in the middle to reveal a four-chamber secret compartment for .22 caliber bullets which could be shot out of a protruding fake aerial.

"These would be lethal at 10 meters," said Michel Lavaud, head of a local police brigade.

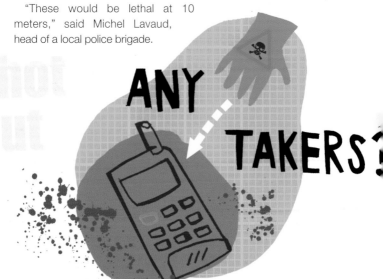

ANY TAKERS?

West Coast Awash In Nike Shoes

SEATTLE   REUTERS

They may be wet, even a bit briny, and it might be hard to find a matching pair, but you won't find Nike Inc. shoes cheaper anywhere.

The maker of athletic gear lost 45,756 shoes—or 22,878 pairs—that fell off a storm-tossed container ship in December on the way from Long Beach, California, to Tacoma, Washington. Now beachcombers are finding them along the Pacific coast of Canada and the United States.

According to Seattle oceanographer and flotsam buff Curtis Ebbesmeyer, who is cataloguing Nike beachings in Washington state, the aquatic parade of shoes should continue to land along the British Columbia coast in Canada and meander to Alaska's Aleutian Islands.

Ebbesmeyer assumes the shoes will continue sloshing northward at an estimated speed of 14.3 to 18.3 nautical miles per day since they abandoned ship near Mendocino, California.

Tough As Nails In The Face Of Danger

HONG KONG   REUTERS

The old Chinese saying "beauty comes before life" ran true to form in Hong Kong this week when a group of women refused to evacuate a burning office tower until their nails were perfect.

"We took the risk because we wanted to get our job done," the owner of the Fingertrix nail salon told Reuters.

Staff members were putting acrylic fingernails on to two customers when fire broke out on the rooftop of their building in Hong Kong's bustling Central district shortly after lunch. Scores of office workers rushed out of the building and no one was injured.

But the five women opted not to exit immediately despite being warned by security guards that they should leave.

"I think deep down, we were all a bit nervous but all of us appeared very calm," the owner said.

Happy with their polished nails, the women left more than an hour later, after the fire had been put out.

SUPERMARKET SALE STAMPEDE KILLS TWO

BEIJING　　　REUTERS

Two people were trampled to death and 15 injured in a stampede by a huge crowd which stormed a newly opened supermarket in northern China offering big bargains, an official newspaper reported.

The *China Daily* said 50,000 people swamped the Hualian supermarket in the Inner Mongolian city of Baotou

The deadly rush in Baotou was not an isolated case. When the Beijing-based Hualian chain opened a store in Inner Mongolia's capital of Hohhot last July, 100,000 people turned out and 20 were injured, the *Shenzhen Evening News* said.

And the *China Daily* said police canceled a Lunar New Year sale last week at a department store in the northeastern city of Harbin over crowd control concerns.

nner Mongolian city of Baotou

TOILET SWALLOWS HAND AFTER SHOWER SLIP

MILAN   REUTERS

A guest at a hotel in Milan had reason to be grateful for having his mobile phone in the bathroom after ending up with his hand stuck down the toilet for more than an hour.

The unidentified 65-year-old slipped as he stepped out of the shower and accidentally jammed his hand down the funnel of the toilet as he tried to break his fall, rescue workers said.

Still naked, he was saved by firemen more than an hour later after calling an emergency number from his phone. The firemen had to dismantle the lavatory to set his hand free.

He was taken to a hospital with broken ribs and a sore arm.

dismantle the lavatory to set his hand free

BROKEN RIBS AND A SORE ARM

Cutting Down Sauna Habit As Cold Bites

HELSINKI   REUTERS

Finns have been told to cut down on one of their favorite comforts during the most bitter winter in decades—the sauna.

A dry cold snap in the Nordic country has sent electricity prices soaring to record levels, so the government has recommended ways to cut bills. These have even encroached on many Finns' sacred retreat after a long day.

"The suggested sauna heat is 70-80 degrees Celsius. One hundred degrees, for example, adds up to 30 percent to energy costs," the statement said.

"Many people can fit in a typical sauna, and they don't spend too much time in the shower."

Media have called the winter one of the coldest for four decades. The dry spell has caused water levels in reservoirs in the Nordic region, which depends heavily on hydro power, to drop drastically.

FICTIONAL WIZARD HARRY POTTER

What Do You Expect From Muggles?

MADRID   REUTERS

A woman set her Madrid home on fire as she cooked up a potion in an attempt to imitate the fictional wizard Harry Potter, emergency services said.

The 21-year-old was rescued by firemen and treated for minor injuries, but half her home was destroyed.

The ambulance service said she had told them she was trying to emulate the boy magician, hero of the books by J. K. Rowling that have been a sensation among adults and children alike.

For want of more magical ingredients, the woman cooked up a potion of water, oil, alcohol and toothpaste, local media reported. It was unclear what spell she was trying to weave.

Ten Hurt As Grenade Wrecks Sofa

TIRANA   REUTERS

A poor Albanian couple's dream of owning a second-hand sofa went up in smoke when a grenade tucked into its wooden frame exploded as they unloaded it, an Albanian newspaper said.

The *Gazeta Shqiptare* said 10 people were injured by the explosion in a mountain village in northern Albania, the poorest region of Europe's most impoverished nation.

It's thought the accident happened after the grenade's safety pin was loosened by a bumpy ride from a local market in rugged country north of Tirana.

Thousands of weapons and tons of ammunition remain at large in Albania after army depots were plundered last year during anarchy that took the country to the brink of economic and political collapse.

WOMEN DANCE NAKED FOR RAIN

MELBOURNE   REUTERS

Hundreds of Australian women danced naked at a secluded location amid drought-ravaged farmland in a ritual intended to bring rain.

Organizers from the small town of Ouyen in far northwest Victoria state said up to 500 women danced and chanted in a ceremony inspired by a Nepali drought-breaking tradition.

"We are all pretty positive that it is going to work and the community here has got behind it just so well," the organizing committee chairwoman told Reuters. "We are expecting rain within the next few days, or a week anyway."

The dance was held alongside regional family day festivities, with the women taken by buses to the secret location to complete the dance either naked or partially clothed in sarongs.

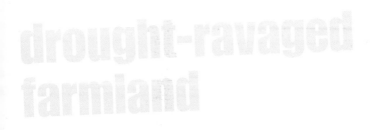